The Measurement Mandate

On the Road to Performance Improvement in Health Care

Joint Commission on Accreditation of Healthcare Organizations

Joint Commission Mission

The mission of the Joint Commission on Accreditation of Healthcare Organizations is to improve the quality of health care provided to the public.

©1993 by the Joint Commission on Accreditation of Healthcare Organizations
One Renaissance Boulevard
Oakbrook Terrace, Illinois 60181

Printed in the U.S.A.

Requests for permission to reprint or make copies of any part of this work should be mailed to
Permissions Editor
Department of Publications
Joint Commission on Accreditation of Healthcare Organizations

ISBN: -0-86688-334-7

Library of Congress Catalog Number: 93-77954

Table of Contents

Preface

All science is measurement.
—Helmholtz[*]

All true measurement is essentially comparative.
—Sir Henry Dale[*]

There is nothing more basic to the "science" of patient care than measurement. Whether performing a history, a physical examination, diagnostic tests, or procedures, the clinician is constantly gathering data to reach diagnostic conclusions and to guide the patient through a treatment course that will optimize the eventual outcome. Each clinician tempers and guides his or her own measurements with the clinical judgments that are inherent to and underlie the "art" of patient care. But the mandate to measure is integral to the clinician's way of life; the mandate is self-imposed.

This book is about a different, but related, measurement mandate—a mandate to monitor and to evaluate the actual performance of practitioners and health care organizations in the application of health care's science and art, and to direct particular attention to the resulting outcomes of these patient care activities. This is not a new mandate, nor is it one that should be any less self-imposed by clinicians and other health professionals. However, it is a mandate

---

[*] Bradford Hill A. 1971. *Principles of Medical Statistics* 9th ed. New York: Oxford University Press, p 6.

that most would agree has been imperfectly executed for the better part of this century.

In the early 1900s, Ernest Codman, then a prominent surgeon at the Massachusetts General Hospital, articulated a simple thesis. He said that surgeons should systematically gather the outcomes of their surgical procedures and care and make this information publicly known so that future patients might make informed decisions in selecting their own surgeons. With his colleague, Edward Martin, Codman played a prominent role in the founding of the American College of Surgeons and in the creation of the Hospital Standardization Program, which served as the forerunner to the Joint Commission.

As a creature of physicians, the Hospital Standardization Program had a clear intent to impose a self-measurement mandate upon the hospital field. And, by most accounts, the Program was widely embraced by hospitals and physicians, and grew and thrived until it was folded into the Joint Commission on Accreditation of Hospitals in 1951. Unfortunately, the strength of the mandate was undermined by the basic infrastructure of the Program. In the Program's final form, Codman's emphasis on outcomes measurement was nowhere evident. Instead, the Program would develop and apply standards, and would use compliance with these standards—an alternative measurement approach—as a proxy for the likelihood of good outcomes. As for Codman, he would eventually be drummed out of the medical profession for his radical ideas.

Assuming the continuing relevance of the standards, the concept of using standards compliance as a basic measure of health care quality was and is perfectly sound. After all, outcomes measurement can only provide performance information that is current to the present time. By contrast, standards compliance offers the potential for predicting the likelihood of future outcomes. This, however, need not have been an either/or proposition. Both types of measurement approaches are potentially important sources of useful performance information.

As the decades of the twentieth century rolled by, both American society and the health care field became lulled into the belief that the latter's own mandate to measure—and to improve—was being effectively carried out. However, there were no systematic efforts to measure outcomes; the standards in use were focused all around, but not on, clinical care and the management of the organizations in which care was being provided; and all performance information specific to individual organizations and practitioners was held in strict confidence. One must marvel only at the considerable tolerance of American society, and of ourselves in particular, in permitting this state of affairs to persist so long.

With the advent of the 1980s, change was clearly in the air. Health services research began to produce compelling outcomes studies that raised important questions about quality of care. And continued escalation of health care costs led to abortive efforts to reform the delivery system which in turn led to rising anxieties about the impacts of these changes on the quality of care being provided. In 1987, in anticipation of the inevitable evolution toward a new performance measurement mandate in health care, the Joint Commission initiated its Agenda for Change. This set of initiatives was designed to place the primary emphasis of the accreditation process on actual performance—as reflected in the standards and as specifically defined by performance measures, including outcome measures.

The intervening years have now brought us to the threshold of systemic health care reform and to imminent implementation of the Agenda for Change. As this book goes to press, the scope and form to be taken by national health care reform remains largely unknown. However, it is a foregone conclusion that measurement will play an integral role in the design of any reform initiative. With the high cost of health care, purchasers and patients mean to know what they are buying and how good it is. And these parties intend to use data and information to select their provider organizations and caregivers. If good data are not available, they will use what they can find to make their decisions. Finally, there will be a common interest in applying measures to objectively assess the impacts of any reform initiative.

So whose measurement mandate is this? Broadly speaking, it is this country's mandate, but it is a mandate that can still be largely shaped and directed by the health care community. In that sense, this book is a clarion call to health professionals, and to organizations in which care is provided, to take charge of their measurement responsibilities.

Why measure performance? We measure performance in health care for two basic purposes. We measure first as a basis for making judgments and decisions. Those judgments and decisions may be made by providers about themselves; they may be made by external evaluators such as accrediting bodies; or they may be made by potential purchasers or users of the provider's services. To state the obvious, informed judgments are always better than uninformed judgments.

Second, we measure as the basis for future improvement. This measurement objective was indeed the principal underpinning of the original Hospital Standardization Program and remains a fundamental integral of any accrediting activity. More importantly, continuous improvement in performance is a basic expectation of health professionals and organizations for themselves. And all improvement opportunities have their initial basis in effective measurement. Effective measurement requires knowledge of what is relevant and important to measure; availability of good measurement tools; skill in applying these tools; and the will to measure the right things well.

As a major product of the Agenda for Change, *The Measurement Mandate* is intended to help health care organizations and health professionals realize their measurement and improvement objectives. In the spirit of the Joint Commission's recent, preceding series of texts on the development and application of performance indicators, this book further translates the results of the research and development activities of the Agenda for Change into practical strategies health care organizations can readily incorporate into existing and emerging continuous improvement initiatives. Its carefully drawn principles, numerous experience-based examples, and thought-provoking case studies underscore and illuminate the intricacies, relationships, and pitfalls of performance measurement.

The text has also been designed to showcase and further stimulate contemporary understanding of important dimensions of organizational performance and the functions-oriented approach to establishing a truly patient-centered framework for improving care and services. To help illustrate these concepts, it provides a full overview of the data collection tools and logic now under development to facilitate implementation and refinement of the Joint Commission's Indicator Monitoring System, which will have a central role in the future accreditation process.

The chapters of this book encompass the hard-earned successes and difficult lessons learned among a nationwide cross-section of health professionals and organizations that have participated in the developmental phase of the Agenda for Change. We gratefully dedicate this volume to their current and future successes and to all those who will enhance and extend their special vision. Ernest Codman would have been pleased and proud of this turn of events.

Dennis S. O'Leary, MD
President,
Joint Commission on Accreditation of Healthcare Organizations
February 1993
Oakbrook Terrace, Illinois

1

Defining Measurement

One of the greatest challenges confronting health care organizations in the 1990s is learning to apply the concepts and methods of performance measurement. Performance measurement operates on the thesis that objective performance data about important governance, management, clinical, and support systems—generated through the application of performance measures or indicators—can and should be used to identify performance variations. Analyses of these variations will commonly lead to identifying opportunities for improvement in the quality of organizational services.

For many years, health professionals have struggled to develop effective performance measurement systems that provide accurate, complete, and relevant quality-of-care data that are useful in improvement efforts. For example, the end-results (outcomes) measurement system proposed by Dr Ernest Codman in the early 1900s was considered by the fledgling Hospital Standardization Committee of the American College of Surgeons.[1-2] The Minimum Standard, however, was drafted and adopted instead (see Appendix A). It established professional support *structures*, such as the medical staff, and held organizations to certain standards of self-surveillance by requiring the monitoring of specified *processes*, such as holding monthly medical staff meetings and "reviewing clinical experience." A professional or public mandate for measuring and divulging the *outcomes* of care, as proposed by Codman, did not develop.

The main purpose of the original structural and process-oriented standards and their numerous descendant standards was to increase organizations' potential for providing services of high quality. For example, the expectation that physicians who practice in a hospital be organized as a medical staff with certain "quality assurance" responsibilities was intended to increase the probability that services of high quality would be provided.

The degree to which services of high quality actually resulted—reflected, in part, by the achievement of desired outcomes as a consequence of these structures and processes being in place—was not, however, systematically and uniformly examined by most organizations. Until recently, most health care organizations believed, and the public generally accepted, that procedures, safeguards, and control devices designed to "assure" quality were in place and worked most of the time.

Today the health care environment has dramatically changed. High health care costs, changing payment incentives, increasing public sophistication, and new doubts about the actual quality of care being provided have combined to seed a growing public demand for actual data or measurements of organizational performance. Substantial advances in information technology provide an important means for performance measurement. For patients and other potential consumers of health care services, the information need lies beyond the bottom-line judgments of accrediting bodies or of licensure or certification agencies.

Many consumers wish to make health care purchasing decisions based on information derived from measurement. Coupled with this need is the recognition that one cannot presume care of high quality always results simply because the capacity to provide that care exists. Rather, organizations must now measure their actual level of performance as a means of demonstrating the quality of service they are supposed to be capable of delivering.

Characterizing Measurement

Measurement refers to the *process* of quantification—that is, determining that attribute of a person, an activity, or a thing (for example, an object, an event, or a phenomenon) by which it is greater or less than some other person, activity, or thing (see Table 1). Each time a patient's blood pressure or temperature is taken, for example, a measuring process is being performed. Each time an organization calculates its success rate for women with attempted vaginal delivery after previous cesarean sections, a measuring process is being performed.*

Measurement has a second meaning: This is the *number* resulting from the process of quantification.[3] A patient's blood pressure of 190/120 mm Hg and respirations of 20 breaths per minute are, for example, two measurements. The number of inpatients who receive warfarin or intravenous therapeutic heparin and also receive vitamin K, protamine sulfate, or fresh frozen plasma is a measurement.†

Measurement then is a word that can describe a process *and* an outcome of a process. When this distinction is understood, the meaning of measurement can usually be deduced from the context in which the word is used. "Make a measurement" and "take a measurement" refer to the process of measuring or quantifying something. "What measurement did you obtain?" and "that measurement cannot be accurate" refer to the result or outcome of a measuring or quantification process.

Measurement permits the conversion of important attributes of people, activities, or things into forms capable of being quantified. Length, temperature, volume, and area are examples of such quantifiable attributes. How long is the piece of cloth? The length (an attribute of the piece of cloth) is five yards (a quantification of the attribute). How anemic is the patient? What is his hemoglobin concentration? His hemoglobin concentration (an attribute of the patient) is 10 grams per deciliter (a quantification of the attribute). How long on average do patients wait to see their practitioner? The

---

* The Joint Commission Obstetrical Care Indicator Development Task Force developed the following indicator, which is currently in the beta phase of field testing: "inpatients with attempted vaginal birth after cesarean section (VBAC), subcategorized by success or failure."

† The Joint Commission Medication Use Indicator Development Task Force developed the following indicator, which is currently in the beta phase of field testing: "inpatients receiving warfarin or intravenous therapeutic heparin who also receive vitamin K, protamine sulfate, or fresh frozen plasma."

Table 1

Definitions of *Measurement,*
Indicator, Performance Measure,
and *Unit of Measure*

Measurement:	1. Process of quantification; 2. Number resulting from the quantification process.
Indicator:	1. A valid and reliable quantitative process or outcome measure related to one or more dimensions of performance such as effectiveness and appropriateness. 2. A statistical value that provides an indication of the condition or direction over time of an organization's performance of a specified process, or an organization's achievement of a specified outcome. For example, in most hospitals, a primary cesarean section rate of 32% is an indicator of the organization's need to further investigate this process of care.
Performance measure:	1. Any device for measuring (quantifying) level of performance. 2. An objective measure that may be used as an indicator of, say, quality.
Unit of measure:	A defined amount of an attribute of a person, an activity, or a thing (such as an event, an object, or a phenomenon); for example, a Fahrenheit degree (a unit of measure) is a defined amount of the heat (an attribute) of an oven (an object), or:
	Fahrenheit degree = unit of measure
	heat = the attribute a degree measures
	oven = object bearing the attribute.

average time (an attribute of the process) is 20 minutes (a quantification of the attribute).

The conversion of attributes into forms capable of being quantified is accomplished in three steps. First, a unit of measure must be defined; second, a measurement instrument, calibrated in terms of the unit of measure, is devised and validated; and third, the measurement instrument is applied to the object being measured to quantify the attribute expressed by the unit of measure.

Defining Unit of Measure

A *unit of measure* (see Table 1) is a defined amount of an attribute of a person, an activity, or a thing (such as an event, an object, or a phenomenon). Consider the previously posited question: "How long is the piece of cloth?" The length is the attribute of the piece of cloth that is being measured. Five yards is the quantification of the attribute. *The yard is the unit of measure.* Similarly, consider the question, "How anemic is the patient?" The hemoglobin concentration is the attribute of the patient being measured. Ten grams per deciliter is the quantification of the attribute. *Gram per deciliter is the unit of measure.* Consider again the question, "How long on average do patients wait to see their practitioner?" The average length of time is the attribute of the process being measured. Twenty minutes is the quantification of the attribute. *The minute is the unit of measure.*

Customary units of measure include the Fahrenheit degree (a unit of temperature); inches, feet, yards, and miles (units of length); fluid ounces, cups, pints, quarts, and gallons (units of capacity and weight); and seconds, minutes, hours, days, weeks, years, and centuries (units of time). A Fahrenheit-degree unit of measure permits conversion of the temperature attribute into a form capable of being quantified. A yard unit of measure permits conversion of the length attribute into a form that can be easily quantified. A year unit of measure permits conversion of the concept of time into a form that is quantifiable.

There are often different systems of units of measure for the same attribute. For example, the units of measure most often used for length, weight, and temperature in the United States are the yard, pound, and Fahrenheit degree, respectively. In Europe and elsewhere, the most common corresponding units of measure are the meter, kilogram, and Celsius degree. Thermodynamic temperature in the Système International d'Unités or SI System of units of measure is expressed in Kelvin rather than Celsius or Fahrenheit degrees.[3]

A unit of measure can express the *relationship of two or more attributes of a person, an activity, or a thing.* This relationship is typically depicted in ratio form: One attribute is the numerator and the other is the denominator.

A ratio-type unit of measure familiar to most Americans is the fuel efficiency of an automobile, truck, or other vehicle. The unit of measure that expresses the fuel efficiency of vehicles is actually a ratio of two separate attributes of a vehicle—that is, the distance (attribute #1) traveled by the vehicle and the volume (attribute #2) of fuel used by the vehicle. The unit of measure for attribute #1 is *the mile.* The unit of measure for attribute #2 is *the gallon.* The complex attribute—fuel efficiency—being measured is expressed by the following ratio-type unit of measure:

Attribute to Be Measured	Unit of Measure Expressed as Ratio of Two Attributes
Fuel efficiency $=$	$\dfrac{\text{miles (distance attribute)}}{\text{gallon (volume attribute)}};$

for example,

$$\text{Fuel efficiency of x brand car} = \frac{30 \text{ miles}}{1 \text{ gallon of gasoline}}.$$

Or consider a person's heart rate, another ratio-type unit of measure. Heart rate is expressed in heart contractions per minute—that is,

Attribute to Be Measured	Unit of Measure Expressed as Ratio of Two Attributes
Heart rate $=$	$\dfrac{\text{contractions (action attribute)}}{\text{minute (time attribute)}};$

for example;

$$\text{Heart rate of patient with chest pain} = \frac{30 \text{ contractions}}{\text{minute}}.$$

Units of measure such as miles per gallon and heart contractions per minute can be extremely useful for comparing attributes between two or more people, activities, or things. Miles per gallon, for example, is a unit of measure frequently used by customers to compare automobile or truck makes. Customers often use fuel efficiency data for many reasons, such as guiding their decision as to which vehicle to purchase. Miles per gallon is also used to compare observed with expected fuel efficiency.

Similarly, an individual's heart rate is compared with normative data by a practitioner or other individual to determine that individual's heart rate performance. A significant discrepancy between observed and expected heart rate may trigger further questions and investigations. An observed heart rate of 30 contractions per minute with hypotension in the individual complaining of chest pain, for instance, usually triggers a number of actions directed at improving cardiovascular functioning. The use of measurement data for comparative purposes is described later in more detail.

Health Care Applications of Measurement Theory

There are many applications of the concepts of attributes and their corresponding units of measure in health care. Some patient-specific examples such as the measurement of hemoglobin concentration and body temperature have been mentioned. The subject matter of this book is primarily directed, however, *toward applications of measurement theory to the performance of organizations and practitioners.*

An important attribute recognized by patients, payers, and other users of health care services is, for instance, the appropriateness with which an organization or a practitioner performs a service. What is performance appropriateness? From the perspective of the Joint Commission, *appropriateness* is the degree to which the care/intervention provided is relevant to the patient's clinical needs, given the current state of knowledge.[4]

Suppose that an organization wants to measure the appropriateness with which the following desirable process is performed: determining aminoglycoside serum concentrations or levels of inpatients receiving specified parenteral aminoglycosides.* The rationale behind selecting this attribute is that aminoglycosides can cause renal damage and therefore should be given in doses *just sufficient* to provide peak levels of 8 to 10 micrograms/milliliter for life-threatening infections and 5 to 8 micrograms/milliliter for less severe infections.[5-9] Inpatients with compromised renal function may require lower doses of these drugs. Measurement of serum aminoglycoside levels provides essential information necessary to individualize the therapeutic regimen.

The attribute here is organizational performance relating to the appropriate ordering of aminoglycoside serum levels for patients receiving specified parenteral aminoglycosides. The unit of measure is *the inpatient* who receives a specified parenteral aminoglycoside and whose serum aminoglycoside level is quantified.

Quantification of the attribute achieves more meaning when the number of inpatients receiving specified parenteral aminoglycosides, whose serum aminoglycoside levels are quantified, is compared to the total number of inpatients receiving parenteral aminoglycosides. This relationship is depicted in the following proportion where the numerator is a subset of the denominator:

$$\frac{\text{Total number of inpatients receiving specified parenteral aminoglycosides, whose aminoglycoside serum levels are quantified}}{\text{Total number of inpatients receiving specified parenteral aminoglycosides}}.$$

---

* The Joint Commission Medication Use Indicator Development Task Force developed the following indicator, which is currently in the beta phase of field testing: "inpatients receiving parenteral aminoglycosides who have a measured aminoglycoside serum level."

In actual numbers, this proportion and rate or percentage might look like the following:

$$\frac{\text{25 inpatients receiving specified parenteral aminoglycosides, whose aminoglycoside serum levels are quantified}}{\text{50 inpatients receiving specified parenteral aminoglycosides}} \times 100\% = 50\%.$$

The 50% rate can be compared to the rates of peer organizations or norms derived from a reliable and credible performance database—an organized, comprehensive collection of data designed primarily to provide information concerning the quality of patient care.[10] The 50% rate can also be compared to an organization's historical rates over time. If the rate is relatively low in comparison to the rates of peer organizations, for instance, the organization has strong numerical data suggesting that an excellent opportunity may exist to improve care relating to the appropriate dosing of aminoglycosides or, more generally, in quantifying serum levels of any medication (for example, lithium, theophylline, dilantin) that should be managed by serum concentrations. If the rate is trending upward within the organization over time, the organization may be pleased at its progress toward improving this process of care. The dimension of performance appropriateness is described in further detail in Chapter Five.

Suppose that another organization wants to measure the *effectiveness* with which it achieves the following outcome: preventing and detecting endometritis in patients following cesarean section.* From the perspective of the Joint Commission, performance effectiveness is the degree to which the care/intervention is provided in the correct manner, given the current state of knowledge, in order to achieve the desired/projected outcome(s) for the patient.[4]

The attribute in this example is organizational effectiveness in preventing and detecting endometritis following cesarean section.

---

* The Joint Commission Infection Control Indicator Development Task Force developed the following indicator, which is currently in the beta phase of field testing: "inpatients who develop endometritis following cesarean section, followed until discharge."

The unit of measure is *the inpatient* who develops endometritis following cesarean section. The rationale behind selecting this attribute for measurement is that puerperal sepsis has been a classic example of "hospital sepsis" and a potentially preventable infectious process for over a century.[11-20] Relatively high rates resulting from quantifying this attribute may suggest a need for the organization to review its policies and practices regarding the use of prophylactic antibiotics in patients undergoing cesarean section.

Quantification of the attribute is most meaningful when the number of cesarean section patients who show signs or symptoms of, or are diagnosed with, postpartum endometritis, is compared to the total number of cesarean section patients. This relationship is depicted in the following proportion:

$$\frac{\text{Total number of cesarean section patients who show signs or symptoms of, or are diagnosed with, postpartum endometritis}}{\text{Total number of postpartum cesarean section patients}}.$$

In hypothetical numbers, this proportion and resulting rate or percentage might look like the following:

$$\frac{\text{10 cesarean section patients who show signs or symptoms of, or are diagnosed with, postpartum endometritis}}{\text{40 postpartum cesarean section patients}} \times 100\% = 25\%.$$

A rate of 25% for postcesarean section patients developing endometritis can be compared to the rates of peer institutions or norms calculated from a reliable performance database, or the rate can be compared to the organization's historical rates over time. If the rate is relatively high in comparison to the rates of peer hospitals, the organization has strong numerical data pointing toward an improvement opportunity. Intraorganizational variations in rates over time (for example, a steady decrease in the rates of postcesarean section patients developing endometritis) can provide valuable information to organizations invested in continuously improving health care services.

Consider that a third organization is interested in measuring its performance *effectiveness* as reflected by the following undesirable outcome: patients undergoing attempted or completed percutaneous transluminal coronary angioplasty in which any lesion attempted is not dilated.[*] The rationale behind measuring this organizational attribute is that failure to dilate an occluded vessel derives from a number of factors including the skill of the practitioner performing the procedure and the nature of the lesions attempted. Rates of failure to accomplish dilatation based on comparison with peer group institutions may suggest opportunities to improve certain processes of care.[21-24] Organizations that track organizational and practitioner performance over time with respect to failure to dilate occluded coronary vessels with percutaneous transluminal coronary angioplasty will have valuable data and information that can be used to study and improve the processes leading to this potentially improvable outcome.

The attribute in this example is the effectiveness with which an organization performs the percutaneous transluminal coronary angioplasty procedure. The unit of measure is *the inpatient* for whom an attempted or completed percutaneous transluminal coronary angioplasty procedure is performed and whose lesion is not dilated.

Quantification of the attribute is determined by comparing the number of patients whose lesions are not dilated (numerator) to the number of patients who undergo percutaneous transluminal coronary angioplasty (denominator). This relationship is depicted in the following proportion:

$$\frac{\text{Total number of patients undergoing attempted or completed percutaneous transluminal coronary angioplasty during which any lesion attempted is not dilated}}{\text{Total number of patients undergoing attempted or completed percutaneous transluminal coronary angioplasty}}.$$

---

[*] The Joint Commission Cardiovascular Care Indicator Development Task Force developed the following indicator, which is currently in the beta phase of field testing: "patients undergoing attempted or completed percutaneous transluminal coronary angioplasty (PTCA) during which any lesion attempted is not dilated."

A hospital with a relatively high rate of failed attempts at percutaneous transluminal coronary angioplasty in comparison to peer institutions or to its internal rates over time would have numerical evidence of the need for further investigation because of the likelihood of the existence of an important improvement opportunity in this area.

Two of the preceding examples have identified performance effectiveness issues, and one example has dealt with appropriateness. There are other *dimensions of performance* including, for instance, availability, timeliness, and safety. An understanding of the multiple dimensions of performance is essential to measuring performance and generating accurate, complete, and relevant performance data and information in health care. One approach to listing and defining dimensions of performance is described in Chapter Five.

Two Kinds of Measurement Systems

The examples in the previous section demonstrate that organizations can measure processes and/or outcomes. In one example the process measured is the determination of aminoglycoside serum concentrations of inpatients who receive specified parenteral aminoglycosides. In another example the outcome measured is the development of postpartum endometritis in women with cesarean section. In the third example, the outcome measured is the failure to dilate a coronary artery during percutaneous transluminal coronary angioplasty.

In this model, two kinds of measurement systems thus exist. Outcomes measurement systems quantify outcomes, and process measurement systems quantify processes.

An outcome is that which results from performance (or nonperformance) of a process(es).[25] An outcome represents the effect of one or more processes on a patient at a defined point in time, for example, at discharge from a hospital. Examples of outcomes include cost of care, patient survival (or death) following a medical intervention, development of a postoperative wound infection, and patient satisfaction (or dissatisfaction) with an organization's performance in providing care.

A process is a goal-directed, interrelated series of actions, events, mechanisms, or steps.[25] All processes are part of, and may be further influenced by, internal organizational systems, including governance, management, clinical, and support systems. There are literally thousands of processes that are carried out daily in health care organizations. They range from performing a heart transplant to recruiting a nurse or other health professional to order a meal for a patient.

Does a process measurement or an outcomes measurement system yield more useful data with which to improve the various dimensions of organizational performance? The answer is that *both* outcomes and process measurement are important and potentially useful in meeting this objective.

Outcomes Measurement

Outcomes measurement is a long-familiar concept in health care. First championed by such health care leaders as Florence Nightingale and Dr Ernest Codman, this approach has seen its most common translation as the traditional morbidity and mortality conferences in hospitals where outcomes of care are reviewed for individual cases of particular interest.

There are several reasons why the measurement of outcomes is important. First, outcomes measurements, or data, are of immediate interest to practitioners, patients, and payers of health care services. For example, for patients contemplating coronary artery bypass graft surgery, measurements of hospital-specific perioperative mortality are increasingly being sought. There is interest as well in the rates of the specific morbidities associated with this procedure. Corresponding payer interest is driven by the reality that postoperative morbidity (for example, wound infection, bleeding) prolongs the inhospital stay and increases costs. As use of such measures increases, important outcomes are beginning to become quantifiable indices of patient and payer expectations as well as post hoc measures as to whether these expectations were met. A project currently being conducted by Blue Cross and Blue Shield of Minnesota uses outcomes as a basis for calculating reimbursement (see Chapter Four).[26]

Second, outcomes measurement provides information that directs organization attention to the performance of a process(es) that contributes or leads to the outcome under study. Consider that the readmission of a patient to the hospital within a relatively short period after discharge for conditions such as bronchoconstrictive pulmonary disease or sickle cell crisis is generally viewed as an undesirable outcome.* This outcome may reflect the culmination of a variety of organization and practitioner-based processes that are under the control of the organization, the practitioner, or both.

In theory, at least some of these processes can and should be improved. Were the correct medication(s) selected for the patient at the time of the initial hospital discharge? Was the patient educated about the medications and how to take them? Was the patient's response to the medications while in the hospital used to help determine postdischarge therapy? Did the caregivers coordinate arrangements for the patient's postdischarge care? Measurement of outcomes can reveal process improvement opportunities linked to meeting the needs of patients and others.

Third, outcomes measurement permits the setting of priorities for improvement of processes. Numerous processes are performed daily in a health care organization. Determining where to begin in process improvement activities can be difficult, if not impossible, unless there are identifiable outcomes that can help pinpoint high priority areas for process improvement. Measurement of outcomes helps to direct attention to those processes in greatest need of measurement, analysis, and improvement.

Fourth, outcomes measurement enables organizations to measure the effect of implementing one or more process changes. Consider an organization with a rate of unplanned admissions from its outpatient surgery center within one day of a procedure involving anesthesia administration, which is high in comparison to national and regional averages. A wide range of processes underlie this outcome. The processes range from practitioner training to credentialing and from operative protocols to maintenance of equipment. It is unlikely that all of the associated processes are flawed, but more than one process may be contributing to the undesirable level of outcomes. While the

---

* The Joint Commission Medication Use Task Force for Indicator Development developed the following indicator, which is currently in the beta phase of field testing: "patients less than 25 years old with a principal discharge diagnosis of bronchoconstrictive pulmonary disease, who are readmitted to the hospital or visit the emergency department within 15 days of discharge due to an exacerbation of their principal diagnosis."

organization may have a high index of suspicion as to the problematic process(es), the effectiveness of subsequent process changes can only be determined by repeat measurement of the outcomes and demonstrated improvement in the results.

Thus, outcomes measurement can be undertaken for a variety of purposes. These purposes usually guide the specific nature of the measurements as well as their timing and the circumstances of data collection. In the context of evaluating the performance of health care organizations, whether this be an internal review activity, external review activity, or both, it is important to identify and measure outcomes for which the organization may reasonably be held accountable. Because the patient introduces variables that are often beyond the control of the organization (such as severity of illness or comorbid conditions), all outcome measurements do not ensure an absolute ability to establish links to processes controlled by the organization. However, for those outcomes known to follow most predictably from specific processes, proper selection of outcome measures can create a rational framework for evaluating care and identifying appropriate process improvements.

Process Measurement

As an approach to assessing the results of treatment and service, the need for process measurement can be more difficult for patients and other users of services to understand. Most users of services, for instance, will quickly grasp the import of an undesirable outcome such as nephrotoxicity or ototoxicity caused by administration of inappropriate doses of an aminoglycoside.* They may have less patience, however, with explanations of the need to measure the rate at which an organization obtains aminoglycoside serum levels in patients receiving specified parenteral aminoglycosides—that is, a process—that is closely related to outcomes such as aminoglycoside-induced nephrotoxicity.* Process measurements, nevertheless, are important to the effective management and improvement of organizational performance for several reasons.

---

* The Joint Commission Medication Use Indicator Development Task Force developed the following indicator, which is currently in the beta phase of field testing: "inpatients receiving parenteral aminoglycosides who have a measured aminoglycoside serum level."

First, process measurement may be the only practical alternative when measurement of a specific outcome is simply not feasible. For example, the organization that is involved in the care of many breast cancer patients will commonly have difficulty in determining long-term outcomes because patients may move away, seek care at another institution, or otherwise be lost to follow-up. Because the outcomes are so far removed in time and may simply not be obtainable, the organization may decide to measure a process, such as the degree to which breast cancer patients receive systemic adjuvant or radiation therapy, which is linked to an outcome, such as five-year survival.* Such therapy could reasonably be viewed as a proxy for long-term survival because it is known this therapy improves overall long-term survival in this group of patients.

Second, virtually all outcomes can be changed only by altering and improving the processes that lead to the outcomes. This means that the processes leading to outcomes need to be studied and measured to determine current levels of performance and variation. Consider a patient who does not achieve a cure for tuberculosis because of a dysfunctional organizational process for dispensing and administering antituberculous medications (for example, wrong medication, wrong dose, wrong patient). The only way this undesirable outcome can be changed and improved is to study and measure the processes involved in dispensing and administering antituberculous medications.

Finally, certain processes are known to be critically important to achievement of a desired outcome or are known to be problematic. Both warrant ongoing attention and prioritization for study and improvement. These processes tend to be difficult to carry out because of the need for multiple interlinked organization units to work in synchrony to achieve desired objectives. A common problem in many organizations, for example, is unacceptably long turnaround or cycle times for clinical laboratory, imaging, and electrocardiographic diagnostic testing processes. These processes cross multiple departmental lines and disciplines and are especially prone to dysfunction. As another example, the introduction of a new clinical

---

* The Joint Commission Oncology Care Indicator Development Task Force developed the following indicator, which currently is in the beta phase of field testing: "female patients with American Joint Committee on Cancer (AJCC) Stage II pathologic lymph node positive primary invasive breast cancer treated with systemic adjuvant therapy."

procedure in an organization frequently strains existing support processes or requires the introduction of untested new processes. These processes are also prime candidates for measurement.

Measurement and Comparison

All true measurement is comparative.[27] This means that the process of quantification is undertaken with the objective of obtaining a number that can be compared to some other number or numbers to establish a relationship or relationships and provide information that can be used to make decisions and take action. An observed measurement such as a body temperature of 103 degrees Fahrenheit, for example, is meaningful to a measurer because he or she knows that the expected temperature of the average healthy human is about 98.6 degrees Fahrenheit.

The relationship—in this case, a discrepancy—between the expected and observed temperatures, provides important information that can trigger and form the basis for many important subsequent decision-making processes. Is the thermometer, for instance, working, and was it used correctly? The issue of data accuracy described later in the book is important because of the considerable response data can prompt. If the data are accurate, should a practitioner be called? Which patient assessment tools—history and physical examination, blood cultures, chest radiography, urinalysis, urine culture, and/or lumbar puncture—if any, should be performed? Should an antibiotic be given and, if so, which one and by which route? Does the patient require hospitalization and, if so, why? What other needs of the patient should be considered?

Consider a second example, say, that a hospital wants to measure the degree to which patients are successfully giving birth vaginally after a previous cesarean section.* Twenty patients out of 100 patients with previous cesarean sections successfully deliver vaginally during one data collection period. A rate of approximately 20% is calculated. Some hospital staff members may ask, "So what does this percentage mean?"

---

* The Joint Commission Obstetrical Care Indicator Development Task Force developed the following indicator, which is currently in the beta phase of field testing: "patients with attempted vaginal birth after cesarean section (VBAC), subcategorized by success or failure."

Twenty percent as an isolated number may have little meaning to the hospital staff members. The number develops considerable meaning, however, when it is compared to the average percentage of successful vaginal births after cesarean sections—75%—for peer hospitals during the same data collection period, and when it is compared to the hospital's own previous rate of 15% (all of these percentages are hypothetical). The hospital staff members may be pleased that their rate is increasing from 15% to 20% but investigate why their rate is disproportionately lower than the rate reported by peer institutions.

Measurement and Assessment

There is sometimes confusion as to the meaning of the terms *measurement* and *assessment*. Measurement is the first but critical phase in a performance measurement, assessment, and improvement system (see Chapter Seven). Measurement is followed by performance assessment, which includes, among other processes, the analysis and interpretation of measurements or data. The assessment process is expected to establish a reasoned basis for specific actions that are designed to improve performance relating to a process or outcome of care. The reliability and validity of the measurements are essential to the credibility of all subsequent assessment activities.

Indicators, Performance Measures, and Units of Measure

The terms *indicators, performance measures,* and *units of measure* are closely related and frequently used interchangeably. *Indicators* are valid and reliable quantitative process or outcome measures related to one or more dimensions of performance such as effectiveness and appropriateness. An example of a process indicator developed by the Joint Commission Medication Use Indicator Development Task Force is "inpatients with seven or more prescribed medications on discharge." [*]

The term *indicator* is also commonly used to refer to a statistical value that provides an indication of the condition or direction over

---

[*] The Joint Commission Medication Use Task Force for Indicator Development developed the following indicator, which is currently in the beta phase of field testing: "inpatients with seven or more prescribed medications on discharge."

time of an organization's performance of a specified process or an organization's achievement of a specified outcome.[28]

Consider, for instance, that a hospital is measuring its performance in documenting the etiology of congestive heart failure and substantiating the diagnosis with chest x-ray for patients with a principal discharge diagnosis of congestive heart failure.* An increase in the rate of documentation of the etiology of congestive heart failure and substantiation of the diagnosis with chest x-ray from, say, 30% to 80% over time (these numbers are hypothetical), is an indicator that the organization appears to be achieving improved documentation and substantiation through chest x-ray of the diagnosis of congestive heart failure for patients with a principal discharge diagnosis of congestive heart failure. A desirable rate for a process or an outcome is sometimes also referred to as an *indicator of quality*, or an indicator of a quality thing such as a hospital or a practitioner.

Performance measures are devices used to determine level of performance. Indicators and generic screens are two types of performance measures.[29-30]

Performance measure has a second meaning: This is an objective measure of performance that can be an indicator of a thing such as quality. One might say, for example, that a decreasing rate from 90% (one measure of performance or performance measure) to 60% (a second measure of performance) for execution of a defined process may be an indicator (or promising indication) that the hospital is improving its execution of the process over time. Stated in another way, one could say that this specific performance measure is an indicator of quality.

A *unit of measure* is a defined amount of an attribute of people, activities, or things (such as objects, events, or phenomena). Thus the unit of measure for the indicator "inpatients with seven or more prescribed medications on discharge" would be the total number of inpatients receiving more than seven prescriptions for medications at discharge divided by the total number of inpatients discharged.* This

---

* The Joint Commission Cardiovascular Care Indicator Development Task Force developed the following indicator, which is currently in the beta phase of field testing: "patients with principal discharge diagnosis of congestive heart failure (CHF) with documented etiology and chest x-ray substantiation of congestive heart failure."

unit of measure is expressed by the following ratio:

$$\frac{\text{Total number of inpatients receiving more than seven}}{\text{Total number of inpatients discharged}}.$$

Summary Observations

The growing public demand for information relating to the performance of health care organizations has driven interest in creating measurement systems that generate reliable and valid performance measurements. There are several important observations concerning the recent surge of interest in outcomes and process measurement and improvement in health care.

1. Measurement has two meanings: the process of quantification and the number resulting from the quantification process.

2. A system of measurement involves definition of a unit of measure which permits conversion of attributes of people, activities, or things (such as events, objects, or phenomena) into forms capable of being quantified.

3. A unit of measure is a defined amount of an attribute of a person, an activity, or a thing (such as an event, an object, or a phenomenon); for example, a meter (a unit of measure) is a defined amount of the length (an attribute) of a piece of cloth (an object).

4. A unit of measure may also be a defined amount of two or more attributes of a person, an activity, or a thing (such as an event, an object, or a phenomenon). This type of unit of measure is usually expressed as a ratio of the attributes of interest; for example, miles per hour (a unit of measure) is a defined amount of the speed (an attribute miles per hour measures) of the wind (the object bearing the attribute). A unit of measure may also be expressed as a proportion, meaning that the numerator is expressed as a subset of the denominator.

5. Outcomes measurement and process measurement by health care organizations are each essential for a number of reasons. A process is a goal-directed, interrelated series of actions, events, mechanisms, or steps. An outcome is that which results from performance (or nonperformance) of a process(es).

6. All true measurement is comparative. Comparisons are helpful both within an organization over time and between organizations.

7. Measurement is the first step in a performance measurement, assessment, and improvement system. Performance assessment involves, among other processes, the analysis and interpretation of measurement data.

8. The terms "performance measure," "indicator," and "unit of measure" are closely related in meaning and are frequently used interchangeably.

References

1. Stephenson GW. 1981. The College's role in hospital standardization. *Bull Am Coll Surg* 66:17–29.

2. Schlicke CP. 1973. American surgery's noblest experiment. *Arch Surg* 106(4):379–385.

3. Juran JM, Gryna FM. 1988. *Juran's Quality Control Handbook* 4th ed. New York: McGraw-Hill Book Co, pp 18.57–18.58.

4. Joint Commission on Accreditation of Healthcare Organizations. 1990. *Primer on Indicator Development and Application.* Oakbrook Terrace, IL, p 8.

5. Carlstedt BC, et al. 1989. Aminoglycoside dosing in pediatric patients. *Ther Drug Monit* 11:38–43.

6. Moore RD, Smith CR, Lietman PS. 1984. The association of aminoglycoside plasma levels with mortality in patients with gram-negative bacteremia. *J Infect Dis* 149:443–448.

7. Moore RD, Smith CR, Lietman PS. 1984. Association of aminoglycoside plasma levels with therapeutic outcome in gram-negative pneumonia. *Am J Med* 77:657–662.

8. Schwartz GJ, et al. 1976. A simple estimate of glomerular filtration rate in children derived from body length and plasma creatinine. *Pediatrics* 58:259–263.

9. Zaske DE. 1986. Aminoglycosides. In Evans WE, Schentag JJ, Jusko WJ (eds). *Applied Pharmacokinetics* 2nd ed. Spokane, WA: Applied Therapeutics, Inc, pp 331–381.

10. Joint Commission on Accreditation of Healthcare Organizations. 1990. *Primer on Indicator Development and Application.* Oakbrook Terrace, IL, p 112.

11. Angelo LJ, Sokol RJ. 1980. Short- versus long-course prophylactic antibiotic treatment in cesarean section patients. *Obstet Gynecol* 55:583–586.

12. Cox SM, Gilstrap LC. 1989. Postpartum endometritis. *Obstet and Gynecol Clin North Am* 16:363–371.

13. Donowitz LG, Wenzel RP. 1980. Endometritis following cesarean section: A controlled study of the increased duration of hospital stay and direct cost of hospitalization. *Am J Obstet Gynecol* 137:467–469.

14. Gibbs RS. 1980. Clinical risk factors for puerperal infection. *Obstet Gynecol* 55:178S–184S.

15. Gibbs RS, et al. 1981. Bacteriologic effects of antibiotic prophylaxis in high-risk cesarean section. *Obstet Gynecol* 57:277–282.

16. Green SL, Sarubbi FA. 1977. Risk factors associated with post cesarean section febrile morbidity. *Obstet Gynecol* 49:686–690.

17. Miller PJ, et al. 1987. The relationship between surgeon experience and endometritis after cesarean section. *Surg Gynecol Obstet* 155:535–539.

18. Morrison JC, et al. 1973. The use of prophylactic antibiotics in patients undergoing cesarean section. *Surg Gynecol Obstet* 136:425–428.

19. Newton ER, Prihod TJ, Gibbs RS. 1990. A clinical and microbiologic analysis of risk factors for puerperal endometritis. *Obstet Gynecol* 75:402–406.

20. Rehu M, Nilsson C. 1980. Risk factors for febrile morbidity associated with cesarean section. *Obstet Gynecol* 56:259–273.

21. American College of Cardiology/American Heart Association Task Force on Assessment of Diagnostic and Therapeutic Cardiovascular Procedures (Subcommittee on Percutaneous Transluminal Coronary Angioplasty). 1988. Guidelines for percutaneous transluminal coronary angioplasty. *J Am Coll of Cardiol* 12(2):529–545.

22. Braunwald E. 1988. *Heart Disease* 3rd ed. Philadelphia: WB Saunders Co, pp 1336–1337, 1380–1386.

23. Detre K, et al. 1988. Percutaneous transluminal coronary angioplasty in 1985–86 and 1977–1981. *N Engl J Med* 318:265–270.

24. Reader G, et al. 1988. Degree of revascularization in patients with multivessel coronary disease: A report from the National Heart, Lung, and Blood Institute Percutaneous Transluminal Coronary Angioplasty Registry. *Circulation* 77:638–644.

25. Joint Commission on Accreditation of Healthcare Organizations. 1990. *Primer on Indicator Development and Application.* Oakbrook Terrace, IL, pp 10–11.

26. Care Communications. 1992. Minnesota using outcomes in payment system. *Quality Management Update:* 2(2)4–6.

27. Bradford Hill A. 1971. *Principles of Medical Statistics* 9th ed. New York: Oxford University Press, p 6.

28. *The American Heritage Dictionary of the English Language* 3rd ed. 1992. Boston: Houghton Mifflin Co, p 919.

29. O'Leary DS. 1991. Beyond generic occurrence screening. *JAMA* 265:1993–1994.

30. Sanazaro PJ, Mills DH. 1991. A critique of the use of generic screening in quality assessment. *JAMA* 265:1977–1979.

2

The Benefits of Measurement

Measurement of organizational performance presents a new challenge to many health professionals who may question its relevance or usefulness to the delivery of health care services. There are many important benefits of measurement described in the following paragraphs including, for instance, the creation of a common language and the establishment of performance benchmarks.

The degree to which health professionals understand the benefits of the measurement process for themselves and for their organization can influence their willingness to become engaged in the process. Participation of health professionals at all levels of health care organizations in the measurement of important processes and outcomes is an essential requirement if performance measurement efforts are to bear fruit.

The Language of Measurement

One of the most important benefits of measurement is that it creates a common language based on numeric values. Together these values constitute an immensely valuable set of numeric points of reference. The language of measurement enables organization staff members, for example, to say, "Our rate of performing this procedure is 50%.

This number compares to the current statewide rate of 5% and national rate of 7%. Why is our rate higher?" Quantitative measurement creates the opportunity for an organization to compare its numeric rate for an outcome or process to its own historical rates or to local, regional, national, or international rates to the extent that these exist and are available.

The absence of quantitative data, by contrast, consigns people to the expression of opinions based on their "sense" that the organization's rate for performing a procedure or achieving a certain outcome is too high, just right, not high enough, much better since "so-and-so" left, or much worse than years ago. The imprecision and potential inaccuracy of such judgments may lead to flawed decision making and reduced ability to identify real opportunities to improve performance and outcomes.

Measurement and quantitative language have long demonstrated a remarkable ability to focus attention, clarify issues, set priorities, assist decision making, aid in predictions of trends and outcomes, and solve problems in the fields of science and technology. Health care providers, for example, use numeric language many times each day as they measure and interpret patients' blood pressures, serum potassium levels, and cardiac outputs and make a wide variety of policy and operational decisions, such as expanding or upgrading existing services or adding new services, and purchasing new technologies.

An observed upward trend in serum potassium levels measured over time, for example, enables a practitioner to intervene *before* a patient experiences hyperkalemic cardiac asystole. A persistently elevated blood pressure measured over time enables a practitioner to treat a patient before a hypertensive cerebrovascular accident results. Cardiac output measurements can provide information that can be used by practitioners to improve the chances that a patient will survive an anterior myocardial infarction.

Similarly, a steady upward trend with no reversals in levels of utilization of emergency services measured over time provides an organization with data and information that can be used to make decisions about expanding and/or upgrading these services. Steadily increasing (or decreasing) hospital revenues over time in a similar manner provide a hospital with data and information that can be used for many purposes.

The language of measurement is more than a new set of symbols consisting of numbers instead of words. The language of measurement can and does change the way people conceptualize and order their reality. Two medical specialties or disciplines, for instance, whose members are trained to perform the same hospital procedure, may disagree about who is better qualified to perform the procedure. The issue may never be resolved until the performance of each specialty group is actually measured—that is, one or more relevant indicators are developed by the groups and then applied to generate accurate and complete performance data for assessment.

The specialty groups may be surprised to find that level of performance is less related to which specialty is performing the procedure and more defined by other factors such as patient severity of illness; individual practitioner competence; and the quality of management, clinical, and support services provided by the organization in which the procedure is performed. The important point here is that data-based performance measurement can change the way groups approach and deal with issues and problems. Individuals and groups learn that accurate and complete data can provide insights and answers not usually obtainable with more subjective approaches.

Benchmarks of Performance

Measurement can establish benchmarks of performance. A *benchmark* is a point of reference or standard by which something can be measured or judged.[1] The origins of the term benchmark derive from a mark made on a stationary object of previously determined position and elevation and used as a reference point in tidal observations and surveys.[1] Benchmarks of performance can be established for virtually any measurable process or outcome in the health care field.

The verb "benchmarking" means to measure a similar organization's product or service according to specified standards in order to compare it with and improve one's own product or service.[1] A growing number of health care organizations are adopting benchmarking techniques in order to improve their own performance.[*]

Why are benchmarks in health care important? People cannot really know that performance needs to be improved or has improved until they have actually measured it.[2] This means a first measurement is needed to establish a point of reference or baseline number. A second measurement, such as a group average from a database or an organization's historical mean, can aid in determining whether improvement opportunities may exist. A second measurement is also useful to ascertain the degree to which improvement has occurred after implementation of changes. One observer has stated that "for purposes of guiding decisions, improvement does not exist (in any useful way) until it is measured."[2]

What does this mean in the real world? During the course of meetings of health professionals to develop, adopt, or adapt performance measures, certain questions and concerns are often raised by participants. "Why do we need to measure what we do and how well we do it? We already know that we are providing the highest quality services in the world because we carefully select our medical staff and know that these individuals are the best in the world. Measurement to prove that our services are of high quality is just a waste of time and money."

Although initially skeptical, the majority of these individuals soon realize that accurate, complete, and relevant measurements, obtained through identification and application of important performance measures, can provide meaningful information about their organization's, their own, and their peers' performance. This information can help to guide decision making, especially if a large number of other organizations are also contributing data to a performance database. This database can provide averages, baselines, or other levels as benchmarks for participating organizations. Limits of acceptable variation around these levels can be statistically calcu-

---

[*] *Benchmarking*, in the terminology of continuous quality improvement (CQI), means to study someone else's processes in order to learn how to improve one's own. *Internal benchmarking* occurs within an organization. *External benchmarking* occurs between organizations that produce the same product or provide the same service. *Functional benchmarking* refers to benchmarking with a similar function or process, such as scheduling, in another industry.

lated and used by participating organizations to increase the usefulness of the data in guiding decisions.

Benchmarks of performance have become increasingly important to users of and payers for health care services. As described in Chapter One, measurements of outcomes are being viewed as quantifiable indices of patient and payer expectations as well as of how well organizations are meeting these expectations.

Consider, for example, the measurement of intrahospital mortality for patients with acute myocardial infarction, subcategorized by history of previous infarction, age, and intrahospital location of death.* If a benchmark for this measurement is a certain rate, and the hospital's rate is significantly higher than the benchmark, potential users of and payers for cardiovascular services at the measuring hospital may seek services at another hospital where reliable quantitative data demonstrate better performance. Health care organizations have already begun to use their good performance data to attract patients, employers, and health plans.

Setting Priorities

Measurements are valuable to organizations because the data can be used to set improvement priorities. Most organizations quickly learn that there are many more improvement opportunities than can reasonably be addressed at a given time. Reliable performance data can help organizations order and sequence their efforts in improving multiple performance areas.

Consider, for example, that an organization has developed, adopted, or adapted a set of infection control indicators. Effective and efficient surveillance for the occurrence of infections acquired in the hospital, and control of infections brought into the hospital from the community, depends on the quality (the degrees of completeness and accuracy) of data collected from laboratory reports, patient records, patients themselves, and other sources.

After a trial period of measurement, the organization discovers a

---

* The Joint Commission Cardiovascular Care Indicator Development Task Force developed the following indicator, which is currently in the beta phase of field testing: "intrahospital mortality of patients with a principal discharge diagnosis of acute myocardial infarction (MI), subcategorized by history of previous infarction, age, and intrahospital location of death."

relatively high rate of missing data elements for a number of the infection control indicators. Missing data can seriously threaten the credibility and usefulness of any indicator data generated for further performance assessment and improvement efforts. How, for example, can an indicator rate be trusted when 50% of the data elements necessary for calculation of the indicator rate are missing? How many cases are being missed in which the event targeted by the indicator actually exists?

One frequently missing data element is traced to an antiquated and inefficient information system consisting of manually written laboratory reports that are hand carried at variable intervals from the laboratory to various destinations within the organization. Perhaps 50% of these laboratory reports are unavailable to practitioners and others at various times for a number of reasons. Another frequently missing data element may be traced to inadequate documentation in, or abstraction of, patient records. Insufficient infection control practitioner training and experience or inadequate support from administration or the medical staff may be contributing factors.

The organization cannot effectively focus on infection control (one performance area) until it has addressed each potential underlying cause of each high missing data-element rate. The organization must prioritize its improvement efforts. This may mean, for instance, that the organization must devote a part of its initial improvement efforts to upgrading its information technology (another performance area) so that laboratory reports, for instance, are more readily available to those who need them. Or the organization may need to educate its medical staff and administrative leaders about the importance of performance measurement, assessment, and improvement (a third performance area).

The importance of using measurements to set priorities is also evident when the level of data quality is acceptable. Suppose, for example, that one or more "special causes" seem to be affecting one process indicator's rate, as determined through interpretation of an indicator's corresponding control chart where one or more points lie outside of the control limits (special causes, control charts, and control limits are discussed in Chapter Six). A second process indicator's rate is within control limits yet shows a pattern of five consecutive points that lie on one side of the centerline. Which process should be the immediate focus of organizational improvement efforts when resources are limited?

One reasonable approach would be for the organization to focus on the process in which special causes appear to be adversely affecting performance. As described further in Chapter Six, special cause variation is not inherently present in a system as designed. When one or more special causes exist, the output of the process is impossible to predict. Special causes of variation that result in undesirable outcomes should be eliminated by an organization.

By contrast, common-cause variation, diagnosed when points lie within control limits, is a result of the random variation inherent in the process itself (see Chapter Six). There are, however, certain situations in which a process can show a lack of control even when all the points fall within the control limits. These include, among others. seven or more consecutive points lying on one side of the centerline; 14 consecutive points alternating up and down; and four out of five consecutive points falling in one of the areas defined by the outer two-thirds of the region between the centerline and the control limits.[3]

In the second process indicator described, five, not seven, consecutive points lie on one side of the centerline. Continued monitoring is warranted to determine over time whether the process meets the criteria for being out of control (seven points on one side of the centerline). The organization can meanwhile focus its resources on identifying and eliminating the special causes at work in the process measured by the first indicator.

Improving Accuracy of Observation and Validity of Conclusions

Quantitative measurement improves the accuracy with which humans observe and record phenomena and form conclusions through data analysis about the observed phenomena. Ordinary human sensing—that is, use of the senses (for example, sight, hearing) and memory as the sole bases on which to form conclusions and make decisions—is more subject to human errors than when quantitative measurement is effectively conducted. Quantitative measurement is especially useful in addressing performance issues that may involve varying degrees of emotional overlay or deeply held beliefs. In these two situations, human sensing is especially prone to error.

For example, measurement enables one to make better sense of statements such as "Americans enjoy the best health care system in the world."[4] The accuracy and validity of this statement depend on how America's health care system is measured. The statement is probably accurate and valid if the measure of "best" is the amount of medical technology possessed or the overall amount of money spent on health care by America, both of which can be readily quantified (for example, the number of magnetic resonance imaging machines per capita or the amount of the gross domestic product spent annually on health care in the United States).

The statement is probably less accurate and valid if the measure of quality is the degree to which individuals can gain access to medical technology regardless of their payer status or the appropriateness with which abundant and expensive technology is used by health care organizations and the health professionals who serve in them. Both of these measures of quality can be quantified today (for example, the number of uninsured Americans, the payer status of patients for whom expensive technologies are used, the number of emergency department patient-visits per annum).

Focusing on the Achievable

Measurement keeps health professionals more clearly focused on concrete improvement opportunities. Improvement without measurement encourages people to identify improvement targets that may be "vague, grandiose, or outside their fields of influence and control."[2] An axiom for designing improvement projects is "If you can't measure it, don't do it."[2]

For example, many hospitals are under increasing pressure to demonstrate improvement in the degree to which they meet their obligations to serve their communities. Measuring this requires identification of discrete quantifiable processes, such as breast cancer screening, or outcomes, such as the amount of charitable care an organization provides, that can provide information relative to the degree to which obligations to a community are being met by a health care organization.

Fostering Commitment to Improvement

Measurement tends to foster participants' acceptance of—and involvement in—the goals and processes of improvement. This is especially true when the participants have developed the performance measures. The measurement process provides concrete feedback—that is, measurement data—that encourages people to take more active roles in improvement. When improvement goals are intangible ("let's do better") and progress toward those goals is not adequately monitored ("let's meet again in a few months to see how everyone is doing"), people tend to lose interest, and, as a result, remove themselves mentally and/or physically from performance improvement efforts.

For example, consider that a group of conscientious obstetricians wants to increase the frequency with which vaginal births occur for women who previously have undergone cesarean section procedures. Simply telling practitioners to try harder to avoid inappropriate cesarean deliveries and "we'll talk about it again next year" is less likely to result in achieving this goal than providing hard data (for example, the hospital's current rate for vaginal births after cesarean section deliveries is 40%, compared to a national average of 76% [these data are hypothetical]). Practitioners are more likely to examine how they practice, to identify improvements, and to learn from others if they know their hospital's rate and are persuaded that the hospital rate could and should approach a more desirable number, and are aware that progress toward this goal will be measured again in six months *and it in fact is* measured again in six months.

Another classic example of the usefulness of measurements in fostering commitment to improvement involves the reporting of surgical wound infection rates to practicing surgeons. Research shows that surgical wound infection rates will decrease by providing surgeons with surgical wound infection rates. Investigators in the 1950s found that the seriousness of a hospital's infection problems and need for preventive efforts were often not apparent to physicians, nurses, and hospital administrators until they were given quantitative data derived from nosocomial infection surveillance activities.[5] The availability of epidemiologic information not only motivated these important groups to take preventive action but also uncovered previously unsuspected infection risks arising from within the hospital and from outside sources.

Recognizing Milestones

Measurements provide milestones toward which people can strive.[2] When those milestones have been reached, the measurements can be used to celebrate the degree of improvement achieved. Performance measurement, assessment, and improvement can be a lengthy and arduous process. Many of the complex health care issues that have resisted resolution for decades will not easily be solved in a matter of a few weeks or months (although some can). The hypothetical group of obstetricians, for instance, can and should celebrate attaining a rate of, say, 65% for vaginal births occurring in women with previous cesarean sections. Even though they have not reached 75%, the data are trending in that direction. As a consequence, they are more likely to be motivated to carry forward their improvement efforts concerning this issue of care.

Summary Observations

Measurement provides many benefits to organizations interested in continuously improving their performance. Seven important benefits include the following:

1. Measurement creates a common language that provides the degree of precision and clarity often needed to identify, analyze, and resolve important health care issues today.

2. Measurement establishes benchmarks, or points of reference, for performance. Benchmarks are used by organizations to identify potential opportunities for improvement and to determine whether performance has in fact improved and by how much. Benchmarks are increasingly being used by users and payers of services to determine whether their expectations for performance have been met.

3. Measurements provide organizations with data that can be used to set performance improvement priorities.

4. Measurement improves the accuracy with which humans observe and record phenomena and form conclusions through data analysis about the phenomena, as compared with human sensing alone, which is more subject to errors.

5. Measurement keeps health professionals clearly focused on concrete improvement opportunities.

6. Measurement fosters participants' acceptance of—and involvement in—the goals and processes of performance improvement activities.

7. Measurement provides milestones toward which people can strive.

References

1. *American Heritage Dictionary of the English Language* 3rd ed. 1992. Boston: Houghton Mifflin Co, p 172.

2. Kinlaw DC. 1992. *Continuous Improvement and Measurement for Total Quality.* San Diego: Pfeiffer Co, pp 7–9.

3. Joint Commission on Accreditation of Healthcare Organizations. 1992. *Beta II Feedback Report: Cardiovascular Indicators, 1992—Quarters I & II.* Oakbrook Terrace, IL, p 24.

4. Fuchs V. 1992. The best health care system in the world? *JAMA* 268:916–917.

5. Haley RW, et al. 1985. The efficacy of infection surveillance and control programs in preventing nosocomial infections in US hospitals. *Am J Epidemiol* 121:182–205.

3

Potential Barriers to Measurement

Performance measurement can arouse concerns and fears that can result in the erection of barriers that limit its effectiveness in health care organizations. For example, providers may be reluctant to embrace performance measurement because of their concerns about the disclosure of performance measurement data and information. Who will have access to these data? Who will interpret data? Will these data be used against providers? Some providers may feel that their professional autonomy is threatened by performance measurement based on data. Barriers to measurement can be more effectively addressed when recognized by the leadership of measuring organizations.

Concerns About Disclosure of Performance Data and Information

Historically, health care provider performance data and information—especially negative or unflattering data and information—have not been actively shared with the public. The findings of the first hospital standardization survey teams, for example, were burned in the furnaces of the Waldorf Astoria Hotel in 1919 to ensure that names of the 582 hospitals failing to meet the Minimum Standard (see Appendix A) would not reach the press and the public. Many of these 582 hospitals (671 hospitals were surveyed) were otherwise well-regarded by the public. Dr Ernest Codman and others repeatedly pointed out that release of accurate but negative performance information could and should detract from the reputations and business of hospitals and practitioners responsible for the poor performance. Many hospitals and practitioners immediately set to work to improve their performance by meeting the Minimum Standard. The public, however, was never privy to the basic data and information that would tell them which hospitals had and had not met the Minimum Standard.

There are several rationales that have been and still are used to support and justify maintaining the confidentiality of providers' performance data and information. First, the public in past decades has demonstrated little interest in information that has been available to them. The reasoning is that it is a waste of time and money to produce data that are unwanted, and since the public has not been interested in the data and information, the public should not have or need access to the data and information.

Thirty-one states, for example, now require hospitals to submit Joint Commission accreditation survey reports to the responsible state agency if they wish to use their accreditation for licensure purposes. These reports include the numeric performance ratings that are summarized on the accreditation grid, a tool developed and used by the Joint Commission for recording and measuring organizational performance. Of these 31 states, 13 require that the survey report be available to the public. Where Joint Commission survey reports are available to the public, however, interest in gaining access to them has been limited.

The second argument for confidentiality is that performance data and information today are technically complex and either may be misinterpreted by some audiences or may be used in ways that are unwittingly inappropriate, given the nature of the data. Consider, for example, that the potential for data misinterpretation relates to at least the following factors: the precision and complexity of performance measures; data collection methods; coding practices; risk adjustment procedures; social, economic, and educational characteristics of the patient population; completeness of data collection;

source and reliability of underlying data elements; type and accuracy of statistical analyses; and the capability and needs of the user.

Of related importance is the fact that a primary objective for the use of data and information is to examine *patterns of performance,* not only isolated performance events or performance at single points in time. Thus the most useful data are those that measure performance over time and that reflect the patterns in that performance. The degree to which a broad spectrum of public audiences will be able to interpret data in this manner remains unknown.

Third, health and legal professionals hold common fears that publicly available performance data and information would serve as a resource to plaintiffs' attorneys involved in litigation against health care organizations and practitioners. The use of performance data and information *against* organizations and practitioners may result in providers being less inclined to collect the data and/or more inclined to "game" or "fudge" the data. In either case, the use or threat of use of performance data and information against providers tends to inhibit their effort to understand and improve their performance in a process that is most successful when internally motivated. This is the reason why society has through its laws established peer review protection both federally and in many states.

Nevertheless, as the cost of care has increased and as variation in process and outcomes has become evident, pressure is growing to provide public access to provider performance data and information. Among the individual and aggregate stakeholders are patients and their families, self-insured employers, insurers, utilization review agencies, the media, health services researchers, government agencies, professional associations, consumer groups, individual practitioners, and health care organizations. The purposes for which the data and information are sought—often in a form that would permit comparisons among providers—range from health services research to bases for purchasing decisions to individual needs in choosing a health care organization. Some groups, such as the American Association of Retired Persons, not only seek specific performance data but also emphasize the need for useful interpretation of these data— that is, converting the data into meaningful information on which decisions can be based.

A large and increasing amount of performance data already exists in the public domain. These data are of variable quality and are rarely associated with objective interpretations. Many organizations are experiencing growing frustrations with the use by unwary audiences of irrelevant, inaccurate, and/or incomplete data to make important decisions such as where to purchase services. The "honest" organization that measures and shares its performance information with its community may be judged more harshly by the community than the organization that chooses not to measure its performance or measures it and conceals or alters its performance data.

From the perspective of a growing number of health care organizations, the best response to the public mandate for performance data and information is to seriously undertake the development, testing, and use of valid and reliable performance measurement so that the data eventually available to the public are at least accurate, relevant, properly interpreted, and useful.

Professional Autonomy

Traditionally, health professionals have enjoyed and grown accustomed to a high degree of autonomy. The enormous complexity of health care science and technology has driven the notion that only those individuals who have completed rigorous education and training in a health care discipline are competent to assess performance in the application of the knowledge of that discipline. Self-assessment has been widely acknowledged in the past as a professional prerogative and obligation. Even today, patients' inquiries about a practitioner's or an organization's credentials or performance are sometimes met with disbelief and followed by silence or rebuke.[1]

Demands and requirements for performance data and information from the public domain threaten many practitioners who cherish their autonomy and professional self-assessment prerogative. Dr Albert Lyons expressed this sentiment: "The physician is increasingly cast as a tradesman, a 'provider' of health care, taxed as a commercial entrepreneur, put under pressure to shorten his course of study, advertise the cost of his wares, and *submit his performance to auditing by lay examining groups*" (emphasis added).[2]

Professional autonomy exists only to the degree communities served by the profession "allow it to maintain its prerogatives by reasons of confidence in its integrity and belief in its general beneficence."[3] Professional autonomy is inextricably linked to accountability to the public served. When public confidence in professionals erodes, there is an eventual loss by degrees of professional autonomy. As Dr Earle P. Scarlett noted, "A profession cannot force the community into accepting it at its own, or at an even higher, valuation."[3]

The options for organizations that feel threatened by the public demand for performance data are limited in today's health care environment. The option embraced by growing numbers of organizations is to proactively embrace performance measurement so that the public can be issued the performance information it seeks in a form that balances the needs of both providers and the public. Release, for instance, of raw performance data—most prone to misinterpretation by patients, employers, insurers, consumer groups, media, and even health care organizations—might be replaced by release of accurate, relevant, and useful performance data and information that have been risk adjusted and appropriately interpreted by credible and reputable sources.

Negative Attitudes Developed During the Quality Assurance Era

Practitioner experience with quality assurance has generally not been pleasant. These experiences have resulted in reluctance of some health professionals to embrace the concepts and methods of performance measurement, assessment, and improvement.

Some practitioners feel that performance measurement may simply be a more effective way of identifying performance problems so that responsible individuals, departments, or disciplines can be sanctioned. No one likes to be punished or humiliated; therefore improved methods of identifying entities to be sanctioned are met with anxiety and resistance. Acceptance of performance measurement improves considerably when practitioners understand that the intent of organizational and individual performance measurement is to identify issues early, before they evolve into performance problems that require sanctions or result in professional liability actions against individuals, departments, or disciplines.

Another attitude among some practitioners, resulting from negative experiences with quality assurance, is that responsibility for performance problems belongs with *other* persons or departments or disciplines. These practitioners do not see themselves as part of a problem or even as part of a solution to a problem. Delays in receiving laboratory test reports, missing medical records, infiltrated intravenous lines, and many other problems are invariably blamed on some other individual, department, or discipline, when in fact the problems' sources are in *organizational systems* in need of improvement. Practitioners play important roles in many systems and, because they know these systems well, can have a positive impact on improving them.

The tendency of quality assurance to focus on the individual is unfortunately widespread in health care organizations today. This approach fails to adequately acknowledge the reality of extensive interdependencies among units of organizations. Given the complexities of patient services today, few issues of any consequence are caused—or can be addressed effectively—solely within an individual department or by a single individual or discipline. Individuals at all levels of the organization must cross traditional boundaries to work with others if performance is to be effectively measured and improved. The ability to view an organization from a functional, rather than a structural, perspective often requires substantial education and training efforts.

Resource Constraints

Performance measurement requires resources including, for instance, education and training, additional personnel, and information systems. Time, another important resource, is discussed separately later in this chapter. A number of health care organizations may contend that financial straits prevent them from committing resources to performance measurement. In fact, the number of truly destitute institutions is a small proportion of the total, and *failure* to measure performance may be contributing to their destitution.

Notwithstanding some of the constraints in the current environment, health care organizations have been citing insufficient resources as the reason for not embracing performance measurement and improvement since the beginning of this century. Dr Ernest Codman, for example, noted that "nobody was responsible for examining the results of treatment at hospitals, and the reason was

MONEY . . . ."[4] He was appalled with "the majority of our profession who have spent their lives in the practice of the art of medicine rather than in that of science, and, being financially successful, are able to influence the trustees of hospitals against an analysis of results. For years they have deceived themselves into thinking that they were giving their services to the hospitals, and comparison of achievement would be, to them, as odious as a comparison of incomes. They know our results are not as brilliant as the public thinks. . . ."[5]

In the mid-twentieth century, organizations' reluctance to support performance measurement persisted as Dr Paul Ferguson, acting assistant director, American College of Surgeons, noted in his brief to the fledgling Joint Commission on Accreditation of Hospitals.[6] He wrote: "In the business end of hospital management it is considered essential to have systematic audits made of the books in which income and outgo of funds are recorded. When the auditors make their reports, the administrator and board members spend considerable time studying the results, analyzing them and discussing what can be done to improve the financial position of the hospital.

"This is as it should be. Patients benefit when hospitals are well managed from a business standpoint; nevertheless, this is an incidental consideration compared with good management from a professional standpoint. The patient entrusts his life to the hospital and the people who serve in it. Surely an audit of the records of his and his fellow patients' reactions to treatment is infinitely more important than an audit of cash receipts and expenditures. The primary concern of the hospital should be a good balance sheet in terms of progress in saving lives. Yet, how few hospitals, comparatively speaking, make thorough medical audits as systematically as they do financial audits! . . ."[6] A complete transcript of this brief is reproduced in Appendix B.

In the 1960s and 1970s the capabilities of information systems hardware and software increased dramatically, creating the potential for performance measurement based on data. Most organizations, however, failed to explore and develop potentially useful performance databases (that is, organized, comprehensive collections of data designed primarily to provide information concerning the quality of care), citing, most consistently, "pressures to minimize expenditures not contributing obviously and directly to growth or operating efficiency."[7]

There are several reasons why organizations believe that performance measurement costs too much. First, they don't know that it won't—therefore, they conclude, it will. This mentality is often rooted in past experiences where the results of resource investment were difficult to identify and quantify.

Determining the costs of measurement has been an important priority of the Joint Commission during the development of alpha and beta testing phases of its indicator monitoring system. For instance, the hours per week required, and the average start-up phase costs incurred by beta hospitals during testing of indicators for the indicator monitoring system have been carefully measured.

Some organizations cannot afford to support performance measurement because they are constantly spending down their resources to react to immediate problems such as taking care of patient complaints and resolving conflicts between departments or disciplines. As a result, there are few resources remaining to devote to the proactive measurement, assessment, and improvement of performance. Organizations that take a proactive approach can more successfully resolve problems when they are at an early and more manageable stage.

Other organizations have disordered priorities concerning where their resources are best allocated and do not therefore have adequate resources to invest in performance measurement efforts. Monies may, for example, be spent on purchasing and operating a fixed magnetic resonance imaging machine—the second, third, or fourth in a medium-sized community—or other expensive technologies when serious performance issues exist that require attention and resources.

Another reason why some organizations claim resource constraints prevent their embrace of performance measurement based on data in health care is they believe it is "just another fad." Their goal in delaying the flow of resources into this activity is to outlast the fad. They do not understand that organizations are now spending large amounts of money on data collection. The challenge is to redirect data collection activities to well-conceived, high-leverage improvement activities.

The call for performance measurement and improvement in health care has not been successfully silenced since Codman and the American College of Surgeons first expressed their concerns about the quality of hospital care and the need for accountability of health care providers to the public nearly a century ago. It is unlikely that performance measurement based on data is a fad in light of the public need for accurate and complete information that will permit the formulation of effective health care policy in the twenty-first century.

Time Constraints

Time unavailability is often cited as a barrier to measuring and improving performance. This is especially true of physicians whose time is highly constrained yet whose input is crucial to the success of performance measurement in health care organizations. A growing base of experience suggests that the absence of physicians from organizational measurement processes is likely to adversely influence organizationwide efforts to improve performance.[8]

Performance measurement does require time commitment from practitioners and management and support staff members in an organization. The problem is that practitioners often spend time doing support staff or managerial work either because there are no support staff members or managers, or support staff members and managers are not doing what they are supposed to do, so that practitioners can do what they are best able to do. The problem then is not so much that there are *insufficient* amounts of time to complete tasks but that available time is used *inefficiently*. Organizations that complain about burdensome time requirements for performance measurement activities on closer analysis are often using available time in an inefficient manner.

In many hospitals, for example, physicians are not provided with adequate education about modern concepts and methods in performance measurement. The tendency of many physicians to develop sentinel event performance measures that identify the most egregious outcomes of poor care, rather than aggregate data indicators, exemplifies the need for education (see Chapter Seven for a discussion of aggregate data versus sentinel event performance measures). As organizations become more experienced in performance measurement based on data, they learn that physician time is best used to develop or adopt relevant and useful units of measure, interpret data, and perform peer review.[8]

Peer Review

Performance measurement is not a substitute for peer review. Rather, it identifies those areas where the peer review process may be most effectively applied. However, some individuals resist performance measurement precisely because of its ability to better identify those areas where peer review should be focused. When accurate, complete, and relevant data are available and point to an improvement opportunity, lack of, or delay in taking, action becomes almost indefensible. Objective performance data require professionals to meet a more explicit level of accountability—objective data make peer-based review impossible to avoid.

How can objective performance data generated by performance measurement improve the ability of peers to review one another's performance? Consider that the goal of one organization is to set an upper limit of 15% for its overall cesarean section rate.[9] Indications for cesarean section are subcategorized by dystocia, fetal distress, breech, and so forth. Statistics on births, stillbirths, and mortalities by birthweight are also generated and stored in the database in order to adjust for case mix.

One physician with a 17.5% cesarean section rate attributes this to the disproportionate number of patients with large babies that he has delivered. The perinatal database allows for a comparison of average birthweight across physicians, and it shows that his explanation is not valid. The following year, after this peer intervention alone, the physician's cesarean section rate falls to 15%.[9]

Peer review has, in recent years, often been equated solely with sanctions-oriented analysis of an individual's practice. It need not, however, be so equated. In the past, peer review has typically involved a case-based assessment of care by colleagues with the purpose of bringing varying experiences to discussion of individual cases with the expectation that poor/aberrant care would be improved. There is a need to understand that peer review can be, and is, conducted with improvement in patient care—not individual sanctioning—as its clear objective.

Inadequately Developed and Tested Performance Measures and Misrepresentation of How Performance Data Should Be Used

Another barrier to performance measurement and improvement is created when inadequately developed performance measures, lacking adequate sensitivity and specificity, are applied with little, if any, prior testing to determine and improve their degrees of reliability and validity. The use of generic screens by utilization and quality control peer review organizations (PROs), for example, has a relatively low yield in identifying performance problems, especially in relation to the resources required to carry out the process. Relatively high rates of false-positive and false-negative cases frequently occur. Substantial variation across PROs with respect to percentage of screen failures has been well documented.[10]

A second, related barrier to performance measurement exists when data generated by the application of inadequately developed and tested performance measures are then used to determine the presence or lack of quality, even when organizations have been repeatedly reassured by authorities that the data will not, and should not, be used for this purpose. The use of gross mortality statistics is a classic example of this circumstance. These statistics are often limited by problems with risk adjustment for patient variables present prior to initiation of care. They are, nevertheless, sometimes inappropriately used to directly judge organizational and practitioner performance. In these instances, the fundamental error of equating data with quality (or the lack thereof) is committed.[10]

Many organizations and health professionals have already experienced the ramifications of inadequately developed and tested performance measures and the numerous potential misuses of data. As a result, these organizations and professionals may have become seriously disenchanted with any type of measurement activity including a carefully developed and rigorously tested indicator-driven performance measurement system similar to the one described in this book. Education and placing organizations in the driver's seat of performance measurement and improvement activities can overcome these barriers to performance measurement.

Fear of Numbers

A final barrier that may be encountered by organizations is individuals' fear or distrust of, or indifference toward, numbers. "Statistics [numbers] are curious things," noted famed medical statistician Sir Bradford Hill in 1937. "They afford one of the few examples in which the use, or abuse, of mathematical methods tends to induce a strong emotional reaction in nonmathematical minds. This is because statisticians apply, to problems in which we are interested, a technique which we do not understand. It is exasperating, when we have studied a problem by methods that we have spent laborious years in mastering, to find our conclusion questioned, and perhaps refuted, by someone who could not have made the observation himself. It requires more equanimity than most of us possess to acknowledge that the fault is in ourselves."[11]

The important benefits of numbers and measurement have been described in the preceding chapter. It is important to emphasize here that individuals who cannot follow arguments couched in mathematical terms will have difficulty in managing progress in the health care field in the twenty-first century. Mathematician Dennis Rosen recently noted that "all the sciences—the biological, medical, economic and social ones, as well as the physical ones—are being pushed by international assault into more logical structures. . . . Nearly all scientists are following the physicists and chemists in seeking analysis and prediction by quantified logical argument rather than by inference based on qualitative descriptions. And their medium of communication is mathematics."[12]

There are three ways to address individuals' concerns about numbers during organizational performance measurement activities. Mathematics can and should be kept simple, especially early on in the process. Most organizational performance measurements and their interpretation do not and should not require advanced statistical knowledge. Second, most individuals overcome their concern about numbers through education and regaining a familiarity with numbers and their usefulness. Third, organizations should and can identify statisticians and others—either from within or outside the organization—who can provide additional mathematical expertise when needed by the organization.

Summary Observations

Although performance measurement is often embraced readily by health care organizations, the following barriers may be encountered. These barriers often reflect underlying issues and concerns that can be effectively addressed when recognized by the measuring organization.

1. Provider concerns about disclosure of performance data and information are a potential barrier to performance measurement that has multiple origins. Limiting or withholding performance data is no longer a realistic option because of the growing public demand for performance data. Growing numbers of organizations now believe that releasing relevant, accurate, properly interpreted, and useful data to the public is to their overall advantage.

2. Perceived threats to professional autonomy may be a barrier to performance measurement in some organizations. Professional autonomy is linked to public accountability. The public is increasing its demand for accountability through access to performance data from health care organizations.

3. Negative aspects of quality assurance, such as its punitive orientation, can create a barrier to performance measurement. Education in the concepts and methods of a systems approach to performance improvement is one of the best ways to overcome this barrier.

4. Resource constraints in the vast majority of health care organizations are, for various reasons, more relative than absolute.

5. Time unavailability is a barrier to performance measurement efforts that can often be resolved by increasing the efficiency with which time is used.

6. The process of peer review, sometimes viewed as a barrier to performance measurement, can actually be improved by performance measurement.

7. Prior experience with inadequately developed and tested performance measures and misrepresentation of how performance data should be used can contribute to the resistance of health care organizations and practitioners to performance measurement and improvement activities.

8. Fear of numbers is a barrier that can usually be overcome by keeping performance measurements simple and educating or reeducating staff members on how to use numbers.

References

1. Bogdanich W. 1991. *The Great White Lie.* New York: Simon & Schuster, p 10.

2. Lyons AS, Petrucelli RJ. 1978. *Medicine: An Illustrated History.* New York: Harry N. Abrams, Inc, p 9.

3. Scarlett EP. 1991. What is a profession? In Richard R, Stone J (eds). *On Doctoring.* New York: Simon & Schuster, p 130.

4. Codman EA. 1934. *The Shoulder: Rupture of the Supraspinatus Tendon and Other Lesions In or About the Subacromial Bursa.* Boston: Thomas Codd Co, p xxiv.

5. Ibid, p xx.

6. Ferguson P. Circa early 1950s. The Medical Audit. Oakbrook Terrace, IL: Joint Commission Archives (see Appendix B for complete transcript).

7. Avnet HH. 1967. *Physician Service Patterns and Illness Rates.* Group Health Insurance, Inc, p 3.

8. Joint Commission on Accreditation of Healthcare Organizations. 1992. *Striving Toward Improvement: Six Hospitals in Search of Quality.* Oakbrook Terrace, IL, pp 224–229.

9. American Hospital Association. 1991. *Practice Pattern Analysis.* Chicago, pp 66–67.

10. Joint Commission on Accreditation of Healthcare Organizations. 1990. *Primer on Indicator Development and Application.* Oakbrook Terrace, IL, pp 2, 75–78.

11. Bradford Hill A. 1971. *Principles of Medical Statistics* 9th ed. New York: Oxford University Press, p vii.

12. Rosen D. 1992. *Mathematics Recovered for the Natural and Medical Sciences.* New York: Chapman & Hall, p ix.

4

Defining Performance of Organizations

The word *performance* as used in this book refers to *the way in which a health care organization carries out or accomplishes its important functions.*[1] An important organizational function is a goal-directed, interconnected set of processes that affect patient health outcomes. Examples of important functions include patient admission to a setting or service, patient assessment, nutritional care, organizational leadership, information management, and assessment and improvement of organizational performance (see Chapter Six).

From a quantitative perspective, this definition of performance incorporates a dimension of scale. This means that measurement of a process or an outcome can quantify the variation that often exists in *levels of performance.* An organization's performance level for appropriately executing a specified procedure, for instance, may be a rate of 30% one year and 18% the next year. Or an organization's performance level for achieving an outcome such as successfully dilating a coronary artery lesion during percutaneous transluminal coronary angioplasty may be a rate of 98% in one hospital and 95% in another hospital for an identical one-year measurement period.

It should be emphasized here that levels of performance, expressed as absolute numbers or as proportions, are neutral—neither good nor bad—in themselves. Numbers such as 30%, 18, 2%, and 5 are only levels. A measured level of performance has no intrinsically good or bad meaning. Those using these data must determine what constitutes acceptable levels and, conversely, the thresholds or patterns that will trigger further evaluation and action.

A definition of performance that includes a dimension of scale makes possible the approach to performance measurement described in this book. This approach emphasizes the need for relevant organizational performance indicators and data and information that describe actual levels of performance relating to these indicators. These numerical levels can be used in a variety of ways to identify opportunities to improve performance and the quality of care. Performance levels, for instance, can help organizations to better allocate and concentrate resources to improve performance and the quality of care.

The Relationship of Performance to Results

A fundamental thesis that drives performance improvement activities is that an organization's level of performance, in the aggregate or with respect to specific functions, determines in part the level of patient health outcomes it achieves. Patient-related factors, such as severity of illness, existence of comorbidities, age, and sex, and community-related factors, such as socioeconomic levels and environmental hazards, may also contribute to health outcomes. Of related and growing importance are the levels of cost associated with the methods used to achieve specified patient health outcomes. The relationship between performance and cost is discussed in the next section.

The linkage between organizational performance and patient health outcomes may be self-evident to many individuals, but there has been indifference and even open hostility to the concept in the past. The story of Ignatz Semmelweis, a young Hungarian physician, provides a poignant portrayal of how performance of a simple process like handwashing improved patient health outcomes—in this instance, maternal survival.[2–3]

Puerperal sepsis was the cause of a 10% to 20% maternal mortality rate in the Viennese hospital in which Semmelweis went to study advanced obstetrics in 1845. The usually fatal disease was attributed to many etiologies including bad ventilation, bad water, improper food, and disordered psychic states. Many prominent physicians of the era, such as the Philadelphia obstetrician Dr JW Meigs, postulated that the mortality in puerperal cases was due to the "justification of Providence; a judgment instituted to remind us of the sin committed by the mother of the race."[4]

Dr Semmelweis, who did not abide by these explanations, discovered during autopsies that patients who died of puerperal sepsis demonstrated findings similar to patients who died of peritonitis. When a colleague died from septicemia as the result of a scalpel wound received in the dissection room, Semmelweis noted at autopsy that the pathologic picture matched that of his maternal patients who had died of puerperal sepsis. He recalled that students went to his ward daily after finishing their dissections and, without washing their hands, performed examinations on the women. He theorized that these students were vectors in transmitting contagion from the dissection room to mothers, many of whom eventually became septic and died.

Semmelweis set out to prove his theory by instructing his students to scrub their hands with soap and water and soak them in chlorinated lime solution before entering clinics or wards and to repeat this procedure after each examination. This change resulted in the lowering of the ward's maternal mortality rate from approximately 10% to 3.6% in a few months.[5]

The initial organizational reaction to the discovery made by Semmelweis was not positive. The chief of service, for example, opposed and denounced the innovation of scrupulous handwashing in large part because of his deep personal antagonism toward Semmelweis. Semmelweis charged that obstetricians, by following the old and dirty methods, were guilty of murder, and he entreated the medical profession no longer to submit women to execution just to uphold an outworn theory.[6] The chief of service responded by condemning him, lowering him in rank, and limiting his practice privileges. When Semmelweis reported his results to the Medical Society of Vienna in 1865, his paper, titled "The Cause, Concept, and Prophylaxis of Puerperal Fever," was not well received. Years later Dr Joseph Lister credited Semmelweis as his forerunner, thereby helping to vindicate the man and his work.[3]

Today there are numerous examples that illustrate providers' and users' growing awareness of the link between organizational performance and patient health outcomes. Consider, for instance, the study that links performance of a process of care—shared responsibility (precisely defined) between emergency department and radiology department faculty physicians for interpretation of emergency department radiographs—to two desirable outcomes.[7] The first outcome is that there is a relatively low overall rate of discrepancies in interpretations of radiographs rendered by emergency department faculty and radiology department faculty. The second outcome is that no undesirable patient health outcomes occur as a result of a discrepancy in radiograph interpretation between emergency department and radiology department faculty. This desirable level of performance is, according to the authors, the result of patient-centered efforts by emergency department and radiology department faculty to support an effective interdisciplinary system of care.[7]

Another study links performance of a process of care—confidential human immunodeficiency virus testing and counseling—with three outcomes: an increased use of condoms, reduced rates of gonorrhea, and reduced rates of human immunodeficiency virus in urban Rwandan women.[8] The authors conclude that interventions that promote human immunodeficiency virus testing and counseling for both members of a couple should be considered in other high-prevalence areas.

A third group of studies linked performance of a process of care—administration of high-dose epinephrine to patients during cardiopulmonary resuscitation—to improved survival, an outcome.[9–11] High-dose epinephrine appeared promising in early trials that were uncontrolled, nonrandomized or nonblinded, and used hemodynamic parameters as outcome measures.[9–11] When blinded, randomized controlled trials in adults were conducted using survival to hospital discharge as the outcome measure, however, no significant improvements in survival were found.[12–14] The experience with high-dose epinephrine illustrates the importance of having strong evidence that performance of a process actually improves patient health outcomes before performance of the process becomes widespread. The strong evidence is obtained through conducting reliable and valid outcomes measurement.[15]

Finally, there is a growing recognition that recommended or expected performance as delineated in practice guidelines or standards must be linked to the results obtained. For instance, the 1992 National Conference on Cardiopulmonary Resuscitation and Emergency Cardiac Care recently published its updated set of "recommendations" intended as "guides for the proper training in and performance of cardiopulmonary resuscitation and emergency cardiac care."[16] Some providers and users of health care services are questioning the validity of some of these guidelines, and they are calling for the establishment of a cardiopulmonary resuscitation database that tracks and measures a variety of outcomes including survival of patients after cardiopulmonary resuscitation efforts have been performed.[15] They argue that guidelines for the appropriate performance of procedures and techniques relating to cardiopulmonary resuscitation should be based on scientific (reliable and valid) outcomes data rather than relying solely on the expert consensus and literature review processes to periodically revise recommendations.[15, 17–18]

This same message was articulated early on in the Joint Commission's indicator development process when the issue of how indicators could and should be used was addressed.[19] Three of these uses reprinted here emphasize the importance of linking performance guidelines development and use to outcomes achieved. That is to say, "performance indicators may be used to guide development of guidelines and standards. Sometimes, for example, valid practice guidelines cannot be developed a priori for certain conditions or diseases because there is a lack of knowledge or expert consensus as to what constitutes appropriate and effective care for them. In these instances, indicators can be developed and used to assess which course(s) of action results in the desired outcomes.

"Performance indicators may also be used to refine guidelines and standards. It may be discovered through use of indicators, for example, that guidelines, developed through expert consensus and literature review processes, may not actually result in better outcomes as had been anticipated. For example, a certain treatment may be recommended instead of another for a given condition. An indicator developed to assess patient outcomes for each of the treatments may show no significant difference in outcomes, thereby suggesting that the guideline requires modification.

"Advances in medical knowledge may require that guidelines, or standards, and indicators be modified to reflect these advances, based on newer outcomes performance data. For example, a new technology may be introduced that produces better outcomes than did previous technologies. In this instance guidelines or standards and indicators may require modification to reflect the advance in medical technology."[19]

The Relationship Between Performance and Cost

Victor Fuchs has recently written that there are really only three ways to contain health care costs in the United States.[20] Each way involves an understanding of the linkage between performance and cost, and "each approach to cost containment requires pain if there is to be any gain." The three routes to lowering costs are to reduce performance of services, perform services with fewer resources, or cut the prices paid for performing the services.

Cutbacks in the performance of services, Fuchs argues, mean that some individuals and groups must receive fewer services. This will undoubtedly cause a great deal of consternation and pain among the elderly, military veterans, asthma sufferers, and virtually every group of potential users of services, however configured, who generally are seeking *more,* not fewer, services. Fuchs reasons that cost cutting is intended to help society; but society as a whole does not consume health care. Rather, services are provided to particular individuals and groups by particular individuals and organizations. Patients are not the only group likely to resist a cut in the services they need. Providers are also likely to resist reductions in performance of services because of "their desire to use their hard-won technical skills and their desire to preserve their incomes."[20]

Improvements in performance efficiency is a popular route to containing the costs of health care. There is a growing awareness among organizations, especially since the advent of the prospective payment system and the application of other fixed payment systems, that the manner in which a function is performed can strongly affect cost. Many organizations have discovered that performance inefficiencies may actually result in higher levels of cost.

Organizations have found numerous opportunities to improve outcomes and at the same time lower cost by reducing waste, duplication, and error. For instance, one hospital discovered that it was losing more than $1,000 on each patient who underwent a major joint replacement procedure.[21] After studying the related processes, the organization identified several factors that appeared to contribute to an increased level of cost.

One important factor was that patients, on average, spent ten days in the hospital following major joint replacement surgery because tests, rehabilitation therapy, and posthospital care for many of these patients had not been scheduled in advance of hospital admission. Failure to plan adequately for patients' needs resulted in patients remaining hospitalized until facilities became available. There was a corresponding increase in cost of services for the increased length of (unnecessary) hospitalization. When the organization began to arrange tests, rehabilitation therapy, and posthospital care *prior* to hospitalization, the length of stay decreased, on average, from ten days to five days.[21] Also, by discharging patients earlier, the risk of iatrogenic disease and injury was reduced.

Another hospital focused efforts on decreasing length of stay for patients having open-heart surgery.[22] The impetus for this effort came from major purchasers who told the hospital that its outcomes for cardiovascular procedures were "good" but that its "prices were too high." One factor identified by the hospital cardiovascular team that could have a favorable effect on level of performance and also decrease length of stay and cost was earlier endotracheal extubation. Open-heart surgery patients typically remained intubated at least overnight, thereby increasing their length of stay in the intensive care unit.

It became apparent that if patients could be safely extubated earlier, length of stay in the intensive care unit and its attendant costs could be reduced. The hospital was able to demonstrate that outcomes were not adversely affected for selected patients who were extubated immediately after surgery and transferred from the intensive care unit on the first postoperative day. Although some physicians were at first skeptical of early extubation, the early extubation rate increased from less than 2% to 25% of patients in one year. More than half of the patients were transferred out of the intensive care unit on their first postoperative day, resulting in a decrease of 14.2 hours of nursing care per patient. Patients who were extubated earlier and their families were more satisfied with the care.[22]

While it may be desirable to reduce costs by increasing efficiency, there may be unacceptable downsides, and this approach may cause pain to someone. Consider, for instance, the increased inconvenience for patients who must wait in line for elective procedures to be performed; who are discharged from the hospital earlier than they or their families want; or who are required to travel to another city to obtain certain services previously offered in their own towns.[20]

Fuchs' final point about the relationship between cost and performance involves cutting prices paid to resources responsible for the performance of services as an approach to containing health care costs. This approach is likely to be unpopular with a large number of Americans whose livelihood depends on performing health care services. Such reductions, he posits, "may also have negative effects on some patients through changes in the behavior of physicians or in the research activities of the drug companies."[20]

In summary, the close relationship between cost and performance of services suggests that achieving a successful outcome in containing spending must come from multiple sources, and "careful assessment of the only three possible ways to contain spending shows that if there is no pain there will be no gain."[20]

The Relationship Between Performance and Quality

Many attempts have been made to define quality in health care. In 1986 the development of a definition was one of the first tasks undertaken by the Institute of Medicine study committee charged by the United States Congress with designing a strategy for quality review and assurance in Medicare (Omnibus Budget Reconciliation Act of 1986).[23] The driving force behind development of a universal definition was the feeling that "discussions about quality assurance strategies have been shaped (and sometimes complicated) by definitions of quality of care."[24]

Institute of Medicine staff members solicited quality-of-care definitions from public hearing testimony, site visits to health care organizations, focus groups, and the literature; a paper was also commissioned to explore the topic.[25] This process yielded 100 definitions, many of which are reprinted elsewhere.[26] Based on the work performed by the Institute of Medicine study committee, the following definition evolved:

> Quality of care is the degree to which health services for individuals and populations increase the likelihood of desired health outcomes and are consistent with current professional knowledge.[27]

This definition of quality and many others similar to it raise important questions. Who decides whether health services have increased the likelihood that desired health outcomes will occur? What are desired outcomes, and are these universally agreed on? How are quality judgments made? Who makes decisions as to whether health care services provided are consistent with current professional knowledge?

The answers to these questions lie in the basic recognition that assessment of the level of quality is a subjective judgment or perception that is made by patients, purchasers, providers, and any other interested individual or group. *Quality of care is a judgment shaped by interests of the individual or group making the judgment.* Quality judgments may be based on a variety of inputs ranging from perceived levels of physician compassion to hard performance data that compare patient health outcomes and costs across hospitals and time.

Performance, in contrast to quality, is something an organization does, as in processes, or achieves, as in outcomes. As such, performance can be quantitatively measured and then compared with other similar measurements. Accurate, complete, and relevant performance data can provide users of organizational services with objective evidence on which quality judgments can be based.

It is important to recognize that different parties may make different judgments about quality using the same performance data. Performance levels are neutral numbers to which qualitative meaning is attached, ideally after the performance data have been properly evaluated.

Consider the variety of judgments that can be made about a procedure rate of 50% for a given condition, risk-adjusted for patient-based factors such as severity of illness, at hypothetical Hospital A. From the perspective of Hospital A, its procedure rate of

50% may be clear evidence of the high quality of services it provides because practitioners continuously improve their proficiency and the organization improves its efficiency through performing a large number of cases. From the perspective of Hospital B, however, Hospital A may be characterized as a low-quality "mill" in which the procedure, even when not indicated, is performed on large numbers of patients to improve hospital and practitioner revenues. Leadership of Hospital B may also lament Hospital A's responsibility for proliferation of specialists who train there and subsequently perform large numbers of unnecessary procedures at other hospitals.

From the perspective of a purchaser of organizational services, a procedure rate of 50% may be evidence of low quality because the probability is greatest that costly services may be being provided when they are not needed. Alternatively, a 50% procedure rate may be attractive to another purchaser that is seeking arrangements with an organization that achieves a high level of desired patient health outcomes and a low level of costs because of its extensive experience (high volume) with the procedure of interest.

A second point is that two parties making judgments about quality may have made those judgments using different dimensions of performance. For instance, the patient who successfully undergoes a coronary artery bypass graft procedure may judge the quality of an organization as superior because the surgeon effectively performed the procedure (one dimension of performance) and hospital staff members demonstrated a high level of caring and respect (another dimension of performance). The purchaser paying for the patient's care, however, may judge the quality of services provided by the organization more harshly if it discovers that the procedure so effectively and caringly performed was not indicated (appropriateness is also a dimension of performance). The dimensions of performance are described more fully in Chapter Five.

Relationships Among Quality, Performance, and Value

The value of a service to users is different from the cost of that service. The value question asks, "Am I getting my money's worth?" "Am I paying too much (or too little) for what I am getting (or appear to be getting)?" The cost of a service may be relatively high but the service may nevertheless represent good value because a high level of organizational performance has produced outcomes desired by the purchaser. For example, a hospital that has a relatively high survival rate for high-risk anesthesia patients may, from the perspective of a purchaser, be providing good value even if accompanying costs are slightly higher. Most users of services seek *good value*—that is, desired quality at a reasonable cost.

The value of a service to users is a judgment based on the inverse relationship between quality and cost,[28] that is, increasingly higher levels of quality accompanied by increasingly lower levels of cost yield increasingly higher value:

$$\text{Value of service to users} = \frac{\text{Quality of service}}{\text{Cost of service}}.$$

Value is a judgment based on quality. Since quality is also a judgment, value is a judgment based on a judgment. The good news is that judgments about quality can be, and increasingly are being, shaped by reliable performance data. These performance data can tell users about multiple dimensions of performance relating to a service and enable users to make more informed decisions about the quality of services they receive and must pay for.

Good performance data enhance the ability of users of services to determine whether or not they are getting their money's worth or to decide between two providers for the same service. It is important to note that even when parties are given the same set of performance data, one user may weigh one dimension of performance more heavily than another user when making judgments about quality and value. Efficiency, for example, may be one of the most important dimensions of organizational performance to an insurer, whereas availability of services may be one of the most important dimensions of performance to the families who subscribe to the insurer's health plan.

In the current health care environment, organizations must seek ways to constantly improve the value of the services they provide to the public. Determinations of value depend on organizational performance measurements including cost. Cost data have been collected and stored in databases since computers were first applied to health care in the late 1950s and 1960s.[29] Cost data are therefore relatively abundant and available, although not necessarily accurate or comparable. By contrast, accurate, complete, and relevant data concerning the availability, appropriateness, and outcomes of care are relatively scarce.

An ambitious project underway since 1991 by Blue Cross and Blue Shield of Minnesota directly links levels of organizational performance to provider reimbursement using patient health outcomes risk-adjusted for patients' severity of illness.[30] If an organization's level of performance reflects a higher-than-expected rate of adverse patient health outcomes, the organization must absorb the related extra costs. If the rate is lower than expected, the organization pockets any realized savings.

For example, consider that two minimal-risk patients (low severity of illness) have unexpected adverse outcomes as a result of a specific procedure performed by a hospital. Only one adverse outcome is statistically expected. The average charges for a low-risk patient with a favorable health outcome are approximately $4,000, while the charges for a low-risk patient with an adverse outcome are approximately $25,000. While the Blue Cross and Blue Shield plan would have reimbursed the hospital for the full cost of treating one such patient, it would have paid only the standard $4,000 for the second, leaving the hospital to absorb approximately $21,000. However, if the hospital had only six adverse outcomes in high-risk patients when 6.7 were expected, it would retain a dividend. In the latter example, the cost for a high-risk patient with a favorable health outcome is approximately $14,000, while the cost for a high-risk patient with an adverse outcome is approximately $32,000.[30]

The underlying concept here is that purchasers want good value in health care. By controlling payment, the purchaser is in a better position to obtain better value by placing the onus on the organization to improve its performance. The organization with a poor record in providing an expected level of performance and quality not only becomes responsible for related "extra" costs, but it may lose the purchaser to another institution that, through improved performance, is judged to be of higher quality.

Summary Observations

There are a number of important observations relating to defining organizational performance.

1. Organizational performance is the way in which a health care organization carries out or accomplishes its important functions. In the context of evaluating organizational performance, important functions are those most related to patient outcomes and include, among others, patient assessment, patient treatment, information management, and environmental management.

2. Levels of performance often vary within an organization over time and among organizations.

3. Data showing levels of performance have no intrinsic meaning—they are only numbers. They have value when used to direct attention to potential performance issues that may require more intense review within an organization.

4. Performance measurement, assessment, and improvement in health care operates on the thesis that an organization's level of performance determines in part the level of patient health outcomes it achieves. Performance and cost are intimately related.

5. One consensus definition of quality of care is this: the degree to which health services for individuals and populations increase the likelihood of desired health outcomes and are consistent with current professional knowledge.

6. Determination of the quality of care is a subjective judgment made by patients and other users of services based on variable inputs including performance data.

7. Performance, in contrast to quality, is something that an organization *does* (such as processes) or *achieves* (such as outcomes) and as such can be quantitatively measured and then compared to other similar measurements to make useful assessments.

8. Value in health care is a judgment expressed by the inverse relationship between the perceived quality of an organization's service and the cost of the service. Perceptions about quality are increasingly being shaped by reliable and valid performance data.

References

1. *The American Heritage Dictionary of the English Language* 3rd ed. 1992. Boston: Houghton Mifflin Co, p 1345.

2. Atkinson DT. 1956. *Magic, Myth and Medicine.* New York: World Publishing Co, pp 201–206.

3. Lyons AS, Petrucelli RJ. 1987. *Medicine: An Illustrated History.* New York: Harry N. Abrams, Inc, Publishers, pp 550–553.

4. Atkinson DT. 1956. *Magic, Myth and Medicine.* New York: World Publishing Co, p 203.

5. Ibid, p 204.

6. Ibid, pp 204–205.

7. O'Leary MR, et al. 1989. Application of clinical indicators in the emergency department. *JAMA* 262:3444–3447.

8. Allen S, et al. 1992. Confidential HIV testing and condom promotion in Africa. *JAMA* 268:3338–3343.

9. Martin D, Werman HA, Grown CG. 1990. Four case studies: High-dose epinephrine in cardiac arrest. *Ann Emerg Med* 19:322–326.

10. Barton C, Callaham M. 1991. High-dose epinephrine improves the return of spontaneous circulation rates in human victims of cardiac arrest. *Ann Emerg Med* 20:722–725.

11. Paradis NA, et al. 1991. The effect of standard- and high-dose epinephrine on coronary perfusion pressure during prolonged cardiopulmonary resuscitation. *JAMA* 265:1139–1144.

12. Lindner KH, Ahnefeld FW, Prengel AW. 1991. Comparison of standard- and high-does adrenaline in the resuscitation of asystole and electromechanical dissociation. *Acta Anaesthesiol Scand* 35:253–256.

13. Stiell IG, et al. 1992. A study of high-dose epinephrine in human CPR (abstract). *Ann Emerg Med* 21:606.

14. Callaham M, et al. 1991. A randomized clinical trial of high-dose epinephrine and norepinephrine versus standard-dose epinephrine in prehospital cardiac arrest. *Ann Emerg Med* 21:606–607.

15. Olson CM. 1991. Emergency cardiac care: The issue of CPR. *JAMA* 268:2297–2298.

16. American Heart Association. 1992. Guidelines for cardiopulmonary resuscitation and emergency cardiac care. *JAMA* 268:2172–2302.

17. Paraskos JA. 1992. Emergency cardiac care: The science behind the art. *JAMA* 268:2296–2297.

18. Kroll L. 1993. AMA-RPS actions taken at the interim meeting: Outcome-based practice guidelines for cardiopulmonary resuscitation. *JAMA* 269:688.

19. Joint Commission on Accreditation of Healthcare Organizations. 1990. *Primer on Indicator Development and Application.* Oakbrook Terrace, IL, pp 4–5.

20. Fuchs VR. 1993. No pain, no gain: Perspectives on cost containment. *JAMA* 269:631–633.

21. Van J. 1991. Factory remedies help hospital cost woes. *Chicago Tribune* December 2:1.

22. American Hospital Association. 1991. *Practice Pattern Analysis: A Tool for Continuous Improvement of Patient Care Quality.* Chicago, pp 36–37.

23. Lohr KN (ed). 1990. *Medicare: A Strategy for Quality Assurance: Volume II: Sources and Methods.* Washington, DC: National Academy Press, p 1.

24. Ibid, p 116.

25. Ibid, pp 116–139.

26. Ibid, pp 130–139.

27. Ibid, pp 128–129.

28. Joint Commission on Accreditation of Healthcare Organizations. 1992. Efficiency backrounder. Oakbrook Terrace, IL.

29. Avnet HH. 1967. *Physician Service Patterns and Illness Rates.* Group Health Insurance, Inc, pp 1–2.

30. Vibbert S, Reichard J (eds). 1992. *The Medical Outcomes and Guidelines Sourcebook.* New York: Faulkner & Gray, pp 7–12.

5

The Dimensions of Performance

Performance improvement operates on the thesis that the ability of an organization to raise the level of its performance and outcomes depends in part on its ability to systematically measure and assess the level at which it carries out its important functions. In the context of evaluating performance and quality of care, important functions include, for instance, admission of patients to settings or services; operative and nonoperative treatment; nutritional care; leadership; and human resources management (see Chapter Six).

Functions are composed of processes, the performance of which leads to outcomes. Processes and outcomes are the object of performance measurement. Yet to simply identify a process or an outcome and begin the collection of data without further thinking and analysis is like beginning a trip without an idea of where one is going or how one will get there.

Performance has multiple dimensions that help to direct individual and team thinking about how to design, measure, assess, and improve processes and outcomes. Human beings can usually identify global process or system dysfunctions with ease but have more difficulty conceptualizing specifically why processes or systems may not be working. For example, poor outcomes may be ascribed to weak clinical care or inadequate resources—characterizations so general that they are nearly useless to improvement efforts.

The dimensions of performance help to dissect and to crystallize these generalizations and, thereby, to direct and enhance actual measurement and improvement efforts. For instance, one person may say, "The medication system is a terrible mess," while another person may say with more specificity that "there is a high level of *inappropriate* use of aminoglycosides in our hospital" or "preoperative antibiotics are not always given in a *timely* manner."

Appropriateness and timeliness are two dimensions of performance and are among at least nine measurable dimensions of performance (see Table 2). The following dimensions are useful in the measurement of processes such as tests, procedures, treatments, and services, and the achievement of patient health outcomes:

- Appropriateness,
- Availability,
- Continuity,
- Effectiveness,
- Efficacy,
- Efficiency,
- Respect and caring,
- Safety, and
- Timeliness.

The importance of these dimensions lies both in their individual and their collective impact on patient outcomes and costs and on judgments of quality and value. Designing processes with these dimensions will enhance achievement of a health care organization's ultimate objective. This objective is to attain the best possible outcomes at the lowest possible cost with uniformly high judgments of quality and value.

Different parties may debate the relative importance of individual dimensions. The dimensions, for instance, may be grouped into those that are primarily related to organizations "doing the right things" (that is, appropriateness, availability, and efficacy) and those dimensions that are primarily related to organizations "doing things well" (continuity, effectiveness, respect and caring, safety, and time-

Table 2

Definitions of the Dimensions of Performance

Appropriateness:	the degree to which the care/intervention provided is relevant to the patient's clinical needs, given the current state of knowledge
Availability:	the degree to which the appropriate care/ intervention is available to meet the needs of the patient served
Continuity:	the degree to which the care/intervention for the patient is coordinated among practitioners, between organizations, and across time
Effectiveness:	the degree to which the care/intervention is provided in the correct manner, given the current state of knowledge, in order to achieve the desired/projected outcome(s) for the patient
Efficacy:	the degree to which the care/intervention used for the patient has been shown to accomplish the desired/projected outcome(s)
Efficiency:	the ratio of the outcomes (results of care/ intervention) for a patient to the resources used to deliver the care
Respect and caring:	the degree to which a patient, or designee, is involved in his or her own care decisions, and that those providing the services do so with sensitivity and respect for his or her needs and expectations and individual differences
Safety:	the degree to which the risk of an intervention and the risk in the care environment are reduced for the patient and others, including the health care provider
Timeliness:	the degree to which the care/intervention is provided to the patient at the time it is most beneficial or necessary

liness). An organization's measurement activities should be sufficiently encompassing and balanced to permit meaningful organizational attention to both aspects of performance. *What is consistently true across all of the performance dimensions listed above is that each is definable, measurable, and improvable.*

The dimensions of performance are applicable to the measurement of virtually all organizational functions, processes, and outcomes, including some such as billing and purchasing that are relatively far removed from the hands-on provision of patient care. The following definitions of these dimensions of performance are purposefully developed in the context of the quality of direct patient care. This approach minimizes the possibility that definitions of the dimensions of performance may become so broad and vague that they are no longer useful. It also emphasizes the need for organizations to continue to focus their attention on meeting the needs of patients and those who serve on their behalf.

The Dimension of Appropriateness

Appropriateness refers to the degree to which the care/intervention provided is relevant to the patient's clinical needs, given the current state of knowledge.

For the past decade, appropriateness issues have received widespread attention in the United States. This largely relates to the reality that inappropriate performance of tests, procedures, treatments, and services wastes health care resources. A large and growing body of literature reports double-digit rates for inappropriate performance of tests, procedures, treatments, and services ranging from coronary artery bypass graft surgery to upper gastrointestinal endoscopy to medication use to hospital admission.[1-9]

One study published in 1992 explores the issue of "the ever lowering threshold for carrying out [coronary artery] bypass as well as [coronary] angioplasty."[10] The authors' study of 168 patients urged to undergo coronary angiography found that 80% of these patients did not meet the authors' criteria for immediate angiography. Of these 168 patients, seven experienced cardiac deaths, 19 developed a new myocardial infarction, and 27 developed unstable angina at a mean follow-up of 46.5 months. The authors concluded that "in a large fraction of medically stable patients with coronary disease who are urged to undergo coronary angiography, the procedure can be safely deferred. While there may be a limitation in terms of generalizing this experience to all patients with coronary disease, we reasonably conclude that an estimated 50% of coronary angiography currently being undertaken in the United States is unnecessary, or at least could be postponed."[10]

Studies have suggested that unnecessary or inappropriate performance is not limited to high-volume, high-cost, acute care services and treatments. A growing body of literature describes similar findings in the ambulatory setting.[11-14]

There often are insufficient performance data to reliably assess costs relating to inappropriateness. The amount of money spent on inappropriate procedures can be quantified only when measurements are made that identify procedures that are inappropriately performed. This depends on an organization's capability for measuring and assessing its own performance. Many organizations have had difficulty with this particular organizational function dating back to the era of Dr Ernest Codman, when the need for organizational self-review was first forcibly articulated.

A growing number of individuals and groups are attempting to compute the costs of inappropriateness from available data. One group of researchers, for example, believes that "few would argue that [coronary artery bypass graft procedures] should go first to all patients with clearly appropriate reasons for their use" and ". . . if society wishes not to pay for procedures in the equivocal or inappropriate categories, then one could almost double the number of appropriate coronary artery bypass surgeries without raising health care expenditures." [15]

Reduction in health care expenditures is not the only issue relating to appropriateness of performance. Most procedures, services, treatments, and tests carry a measurable risk of complication to patients. Patients who do not need a service should not be subjected to its risks.

Appropriateness issues have garnered considerable interest among individuals serving on indicator development task forces convened since 1987 by the Joint Commission as part of its Agenda for Change initiative. The Cardiovascular Indicator Development Task Force, for example, identified appropriateness as an important issue when making the decision to admit to the hospital patients with suspected acute myocardial infarction. Task force members reasoned that appropriate medical care for acute myocardial infarction dictates overdiagnoses of possible myocardial infarction and a significant proportion of patients should be admitted in whom myocardial infarction is subsequently ruled out. However, task force members also cautioned that extreme overadmission of patients constitutes inappropriate utilization (overutilization) of services.[16–19]

The Medication Use Indicator Development Task Force addressed inpatients who simultaneously receive more than one type of oral benzodiazepine.[20–22] Research shows that more than one drug in the same class of drugs (for example, diazepam, flurazepam, and lorazepam) are sometimes ordered for the same indication (for example, sedation or anxiety). This inappropriate practice is not limited to benzodiazepines. High rates of the occurrence of this phenomenon, according to the task force, suggests the need to examine the hospital's drug selection practices and/or the review of medication orders before dispensing and administering.[22]

The Infection Control Indicator Development Task Force addressed the level at which organizations monitor the rubeola (measles) immunization status of their employees and immunize those employees who require immunization.[23] A high level of performance of monitoring for, and immunizing employees against, measles decreases the probability that unwary susceptible patients may become infected with a virus transmitted by staff members.[23–30]

The Dimension of Availability

Availability refers to the degree to which the appropriate care/intervention is available to meet the needs of the patient served.[31]

There is ample evidence that ever-increasing amounts of money spent on health care services have not necessarily improved the availability of health care services to people who need them.[32–33] Americans now face a huge national debt due in part to the inability to satisfactorily "control" health care expenditures. Such expenditures in 1992 consumed $809 billion or 13.4% of the gross national product (GNP). In 1990 national health expenditures grew 10.5% while the GNP grew only 5%.[34]

In spite of the large amount of money spent annually on health care services, their general availability has actually decreased. Unavailability of primary care, for instance, is cited as a major reason for emergency department crowding[35-37] and higher rates of hospitalization for patients with conditions that can often be treated outside of the hospital or avoided altogether.[38-39] "Patient dumping" emerged as a problem in the 1980s.[40-41] The United States Congress and a number of state legislatures enacted strict sanctions against transferring unstable patients from one hospital to another after reports surfaced that seriously ill or injured patients were dying en route.[39]

At the level of individual organizations, opportunities for improving availability typically abound. These opportunities range from improving an organization's telephone service so that patients can call to make appointments to improving the availability of newborn infants to their mothers soon after delivery.[42]

Availability issues have received attention by Joint Commission indicator development task forces. The Trauma Indicator Development Task Force, for example, often focused on developing performance measures that quantify the availability of tests, procedures, services, and treatments to trauma patients who need swift interventions to improve their prospects for survival.

The Dimension of Continuity

Continuity refers to the degree to which the care/intervention for the patient is coordinated among practitioners, between organizations, and across time.

The performance of organizations in providing tests, procedures, treatments, and services for patients in a coordinated manner is an important area that often benefits from measurement, assessment, and improvement efforts. Considerable waste, error, and the need for rework often result from uncoordinated and/or illogical sequencing of services across practitioners, disciplines, departments, and organizations.

Consider, for example, the transportation problem that exists in many organizations today. The transportation problem here refers to a chronic system dysfunction in which patient transportation delays lead to interruptions and delays in important services such as admitting and discharging patients, performing diagnostic imaging procedures, and operating on patients. The transportation department is usually blamed for delays in transporting patients. Careful study, however, usually reveals the real source: the need for improvement in record keeping and cross-departmental and cross-disciplinary communication.

One hospital performance improvement team, for instance, examined the hospital's transportation process beginning from the time a physician ordered a test or procedure to the time a patient was returned to his or her room after a test or procedure had been completed.[43] The team found that the process was complex, crossing departmental and disciplinary boundaries. A total of nine telephone calls were required to get a patient to his or her test or therapy and back to his or her room after a physician placed an order for a test or treatment.[43] The most common reasons for delays in patient transportation were, in decreasing order of frequency, patient was awaiting discharge, patient was eating, patient was in the bathroom, patient was in another test, patient was with visitors, patient was too sick, equipment was not available, patient was with the physician, patient refused, and other.[43]

A key finding in the study was that delays in patient transportation could be reduced by increasing communication across departments and disciplines. One tangible improvement in communication, for example, was the purchase of two-way radios that linked transporters directly to a central patient dispatcher. This resulted in a decrease in the number of telephone calls to a total of four and immediate access for the dispatcher to every patient transporter.[43] Information systems provided physical therapy department staff members with an electronic blackboard enabling them to automatically transmit the physical therapy schedule daily to each nursing station. In this way, nurses knew when patients were scheduled for physical therapy and could better prepare them for transport.

Record keeping was the underlying etiology of the most frequent cause of delays in patient transportation: patients awaiting discharge. Patients awaiting discharge were often not transported on time because nurses had not yet fulfilled their record keeping obligations on discharged patients and were prohibited by hospital policy from fulfilling them once patients had left their units. Patients therefore remained on the unit until charting was completed. This issue was addressed by allowing nurses to chart on their patients up to 24 hours after patients had been transferred from the unit.[43]

Record-keeping issues and continuity of services have been interlinked for many years. Over 50 years ago, for example, Dr Thomas Ponton stressed the importance of record keeping to improve continuity of services. He cited the need for practitioners to record data formerly carried in their memories because the increasing number of patient-physician encounters and use of data-producing precision instruments had already begun to overwhelm the capacity of human memory to accurately and completely retain essential information.[44] "Without a record," he noted, "a great deal of repetition becomes necessary, entailing unnecessary expense and waste of time. . . . All this is reflected in an increased cost of medical care."[44]

Another example that illustrates the importance of continuity between practitioners and across time involves the process of providing emergency department plain film radiographic interpretations. Hospitals are required to provide diagnostic radiographic studies for their emergency department patients when indicated and ordered by emergency physicians, with official interpretations of studies performed in a timely manner by radiologists.[45]

The most common practice pattern for providing emergency department patients with immediate radiographic interpretations— that is, while they are being assessed in the emergency department— is alternating responsibility between physicians working in the emergency department and radiologists during a 168-hour week, according to one survey.[45] This means that a physician working in the emergency department provides an immediate interpretation of the radiograph and bases his or her patient management decisions, at least in part, on this initial interpretation. A radiologist subsequently interprets the same radiograph to check the accuracy of the initial interpretation. Any discrepancy in interpretation is communicated to specific staff members who are responsible for contacting the patient or the patient's practitioner.

This relatively common arrangement illustrates the need for continuity in the provision of radiographic interpretation services. If the process for ensuring interpretative accuracy is working in a continuous manner, the probability that patient health outcomes are negatively affected becomes remote. This means that a high level of coordination and cooperation between emergency and radiology department staff members has a positive and direct impact on the quality of patient health outcomes experienced in relation to this process of care.[46]

If the process is not working in a continuous manner, patient health outcomes can be negatively affected, sometimes seriously. For instance, a pneumoperitoneum—undiagnosed or misdiagnosed by a physician in the emergency department and diagnosed at a later time by a radiologist—can result in patient death, especially if the patient has been discharged to home, perhaps with the diagnosis of "abdominal pain" or "gastroenteritis."

The Dimension of Effectiveness

Effectiveness refers to the degree to which the care/intervention is provided in the correct manner, given the current state of knowledge, in order to achieve the desired/projected outcome(s) for the patient.

Effectiveness issues have garnered considerable national attention because services that are provided incorrectly—that is, ineffectively—may result in undesirable patient health outcomes ranging from patient inconvenience to serious injury, including death. Dr Ernest Codman was one of the earliest advocates of the need to measure and improve performance effectiveness.[47]

Codman believed that hospital promotion systems based solely on seniority were unjust and contributed to poor patient health outcomes. Promotions, he argued, should be based on actual practitioner performance effectiveness, which could and should be continuously measured. Codman attracted the attention of the trustees of the Massachusetts General Hospital by resigning from the medical staff in 1914 as a protest against the seniority system of promotion that was incompatible with his ideas.

On the day Codman received the acceptance of his resignation, he wrote again asking to be appointed surgeon-in-chief on the grounds that the results of his treatment of patients at their hospital during the previous ten years were better than those of other surgeons. Codman had tabulated his results in case the trustees should ask to see them, but since no one had ever inquired into the results of other surgeons, there was of course nothing with which to compare his performance effectiveness. Codman was not appointed surgeon-in-chief. However, the seniority system was dropped not long after, and a portion of the budget became devoted to a performance measurement and analysis system (called the "Follow-up System").[47]

The occurrence of undesirable patient health outcomes attributable to less-than-effective organizational and practitioner performance remains an important issue. Questions and concerns about performance effectiveness frequently become the motivating forces behind decisions to pursue professional liability action.

One group of researchers, for example, studied the proportion of malpractice claims that were due to negligence associated with errors in obstetrics and gynecology, general surgery, anesthesiology, and radiology. These malpractice claims were reported to a large New Jersey physician malpractice insurer between 1977 and 1989.[48] Negligence was defined in the study as failure to provide such care as a reasonable, careful, and competent practitioner would in the year in which the injury occurred. Errors were categorized as patient management (for example, errors in diagnosis or decision making); technical performance problems (for example, improper performance or unintentional iatrogenic injury); and medical and nursing staff coordination problems (for example, problems in communication between practitioners).

The authors found that "patient management (cognitive) errors were the most frequent type in all specialties; compared with technical performance and coordination problems, they were generally associated with greater mortality and higher median indemnity payments."[48] Impaired coordination between multiple health care personnel appeared to play a strong supporting role to patient management and technical performance errors.

Performance effectiveness has been a major focus of all of the Joint Commission indicator development task forces. The Obstetrical Indicator Development Task Force, for instance, argued that neonatal birth trauma and excessive maternal blood loss were both potential organizational and practitioner-based performance effectiveness issues. The Anesthesia Indicator Development Task Force identified the following issues as potential organizational and practitioner-based performance effectiveness issues: development of central nervous system complications or peripheral neurologic deficits during or within two postprocedure days of procedures involving anesthesia administration; cardiac arrest, acute myocardial infarction, or respiratory arrest associated with anesthesia administration; and unplanned admission of patients to the hospital within one postprocedure day following outpatient procedures involving anesthesia administration. From the perspective of the Anesthesia Indicator Development Task Force, practitioners include all clinical staff members who participate in the perioperative care of patients.

The Cardiovascular Indicator Development Task Force argued that performance effectiveness could be an underlying factor contributing to intrahospital mortality of patients undergoing isolated coronary artery bypass graft procedures; failed percutaneous transluminal coronary angioplasty attempts to dilate coronary artery lesions; and intrahospital mortality of patients with acute myocardial infarction. The Oncology Indicator Development Task Force cited performance effectiveness as a potential issue when incomplete surgical resection of tumor occurred among patients with non–small cell primary lung cancer who underwent thoracotomy.

The Dimension of Efficacy

Efficacy refers to the degree to which the care/intervention used for the patient has been shown to accomplish the desired/projected outcome(s).

The need to measure the efficacy of health care services has become increasingly important in recent years as the costs associated with modern technology-driven health care have continued to escalate. Since World War II there has been a virtual explosion of new modalities and technologies in health care including, for example, the discovery of antibiotics, chemotherapy, lasers, organ transplantation, computerized axial tomography, magnetic resonance imaging, and genetics-DNA engineering. Although the efficacy of drugs and devices are, by law, evaluated before release in the United States, there is no such requirement for measuring the efficacy of most of the tests and procedures carried out daily by health professionals.[49]

Measuring efficacy might be easier if the number of new technologies introduced each year were small. So many new technologies are constantly being introduced, however, that efficacy measurement efforts cannot keep up.[50] As a result, new techniques and procedures are often introduced into practice on the basis of inadequate objective evidence about their degrees of efficacy, potential for harm, and cost. Information about the efficacy of complex new technologies is often limited to the personal anecdotes and opinions of a few individuals published in an obscure medical journal.[50]

One important initiative begun over 15 years ago has addressed the need to provide practitioners with better data and information regarding the efficacy of clinical procedures and tests. The Blue Cross and Blue Shield Association began the Medical Necessity Project in 1976, with the cooperation of the American College of Physicians, the American College of Radiology, and the American College of Surgeons.[51] The purpose of the project was to ascertain the efficacy of "new procedures of unproven value; procedures of dubious current usefulness; procedures that tended to be redundant when done in combination with other procedures; and procedures unlikely to yield additional information through repetition."[51]

Measurement of the efficacy of certain patterns of care such as the indiscriminate ordering of preestablished batteries of tests received attention beginning in 1979. In 1983 the Blue Cross and Blue Shield Association asked the American College of Physicians for assistance in a review of common diagnostic tests ("little ticket items"). Responsibility for this project was undertaken by the College's Clinical Efficacy Assessment Subcommittee, and the project became known as the Clinical Efficacy Assessment Project (CEAP). The primary objective of this project is to determine the medical merit of selected practices through rigorous technology selection and evaluation processes reviewed elsewhere.[52-53] Guidelines are developed and published that specify the circumstances in which a test or procedure is indicated, not indicated, or contraindicated.[54]

There are two major reasons why health care organizations are, or should be, concerned about the efficacy of the diagnostic and therapeutic modalities they purchase and employ: undesirable patient health outcomes and cost. Modern health care technology, chiefly because of its complexity and reliance on capital and human resources, is often applied in the hospital setting. There are quantifiable risks associated with most procedures. Consider the circumstance in which problems are encountered during, or as a result of, the application of technologies without demonstrated efficacy. The organization, through its governing board, has ultimate responsibility for the operation of the organization and for providing patient care of high quality. As such, the organization is likely to be held accountable, at least in part, by an injured party.

Inefficacious treatments and procedures are virtually always inappropriate and waste health care resources. Consider, for example, the "routine" use of intravenous pyelography before hysterectomy.[55] Rationales for this procedure are based on its potential for detecting unexpected abnormalities and for localizing the distal ureters to decrease the chance of surgical injury. In reality the procedure "yields a low number of abnormalities; moreover, the findings do not affect either the decision to operate or the incidence of surgical complications."[55] Intravenous pyelography prior to hysterectomy is appropriate to evaluate women with a large pelvic mass or known pelvic cancer. The cost of the routine use of intravenous pyelography before hysterectomy was already very high at approximately $420 million in 1973.[55]

One observer has noted that "the cost of complex, capital-intensive technologies command a great deal of public attention. But simpler, less dramatic, and noninvasive procedures such as clinical laboratory tests, radiographs, and electrocardiograms are a greater source of health care expenditure."[51] Efficacy data and information produced by initiatives such as CEAP address "outmoded habits, lack of awareness of current knowledge, and perhaps unnecessary use in defensive medicine. Much of the vulnerability to defensive practice arises from the lack of definitive information about what it is generally *not* useful to do."[51]

The Dimension of Efficiency

Efficiency refers to the ratio of the outcomes (results of care/intervention) for a patient to the resources used to deliver the care.

The modern idea of efficiency originated in the last quarter of the nineteenth century when Frederick Winslow Taylor and others became concerned with the apparent gap between the potential output and the actual output of industrial workers.[56] Taylor believed that worker productivity could be enhanced by first analyzing and studying a work process before it was performed; then deciding how it could be done with a minimum of wasted motion and energy; and finally instructing the worker so "as to require him to do each job in what has been found to be the best method of operation."[57] Managers were responsible for "scientifically" planning and overseeing this process.

One of the best descriptions of the "efficiency movement" was written by Charles Buxton Going in 1912: "The essence of the efficiency movement is insistence upon a determination of standards of achievement—equitable and reasonable standards by which the ratio of useful results secured to the effort expended, or the expense incurred in any given case, may be compared with the ratio that should exist in a normal utilization of the agencies at hand. Efficiency does not demand or even encourage strenuousness. It does not impose or even countenance parsimony. It merely demands equivalence, equivalence between power supplied and work performed; equivalence between natural resources utilized and products obtained; equivalence between vital opportunity and individual or national health; equivalence between attainable degrees of security and the actual proportion of casualties; equivalence between production capacity and finished product."[58]

Few people then or now would dispute the fact that society in general benefits from organizations that measure and improve their levels of efficiency; more efficient organizations waste fewer of society's resources. Yet when organizational leaders increase efficiency by commanding and coercing employees to mightily increase output without considering the human dimension of work, a pattern of social revolt directed at any improvement efforts often results.

The coldness and dehumanization often associated with efficiency can be traced to the early failures of enterprises to include the needs of employees in their pursuit of improving output. "What seemed to be essentially lacking," wrote Harold Smiddy and Lionel Naum, "was an adequate awareness that the man at the machine might value and protect his own conception of his own dignity—that in the last analysis any hope for a more efficient world would necessarily have to depend on making the worker aware and voluntarily appreciative of the fact that although his objectives and those of the enterprise might normally be different, both sets of objectives could only be achieved together; that is, that their desires were not mutually exclusive, merely different."[58]

Thus was born in the early 1900s the visionary idea that "the individual must feel leadership; have adequate encouragement and reward; be physically fit and under good physical conditions; and receive a definite allotment of responsibility. These conditions apply not only to the operative force but to all grades of employees. In fact, some of them apply with greater urgency to the man 'higher-up' than to the actual worker. . . . Of all the conditions controlling a fine working atmosphere, leadership probably plays the most important part."[58]

The hospital standardization movement, a tradition carried on today in the work of the Joint Commission in conjunction with accredited health care organizations, was spawned at the height of the early twentieth century efficiency movement.[59–60] Dr Ernest Codman often used the word *efficiency* to describe the need to improve many aspects of practitioner and organizational performance. He said, for example, "Up to the present time the public and the medical profession have regarded Hospitals as places for the treatment of the sick, but not necessarily for their efficient treatment. Attention has been paid to the cleanliness of institutions, to the architectural arrangement of the buildings, to the kindliness of the staff and nurses, etc, but no attempt has ever been systematically made to determine whether the treatment so freely given has been efficient. . . ."[61]

Today, finding ways to improve efficiency is rapidly becoming one of the most common performance improvement efforts undertaken by health care organizations. These efforts range from improving the time with which laboratory, diagnostic imaging, and electrocardiographic results are returned to practitioners to improving the efficiency of the admission and discharge processes for patients and their families. It has become commonplace since the advent of fixed payment systems to strive to improve (that is, reduce) the cost of hospital services by improving the efficiency with which the services are provided. For example, the cost of hospitalization can often be decreased if hospital services can be streamlined.

The leadership of growing numbers of organizations today are succeeding in cultivating an equivalence between resources utilized and end results obtained by involving *everyone* in an organization in efforts to improve efficiency. Medical staff, for instance, are more likely to embrace efficiency improvements they have helped to identify. They are more likely to resist changes forced on them by organizational leaders who have not included physicians in the early and subsequent phases of the organization's measurement, assessment, and improvement processes. "Without physician interest and support," says one observer, "data feedback will be the dead end of a short-lived process."[62]

The Dimension of Respect and Caring

Respect and caring refers to the degree to which a patient, or designee, is involved in his or her own care decisions, and that those providing services do so with sensitivity and respect for his or her needs and expectations and individual differences.

Patient-centered health care organizations have a consuming drive to continuously improve their performance in meeting patients' needs and respecting their rights as human beings. Respect and caring is a dimension of organizational performance, however, that is neglected by many organizations today. The degree to which an organization respects the basic rights of patients has a measurable impact on patient health outcomes.

The caring and respect dimension of organizational performance is important to most patients and their families. One study found that patients typically focus on the physician's personality and interpersonal skills as measures of quality—that is, "the amount of time doctors spend with a patient, how much interest they show in who the patient is and in his or her well-being, how much information they provide, and whether they are compassionate and understanding."[63] Judgments about the quality of hospitals are often based on overall cleanliness, friendliness and helpfulness of the staff, and tastiness of the food; patients also prefer going to a hospital that is "*not like a factory.*"[64] Several respondents in the study felt that health care quality had declined in the past ten years because of recent staffing shortages (specifically nurses), less personalized attention, and increased prices.[65]

Patient caring and respect have long been recognized as a major element in the successful practice of the healing arts. Dr Herrman Blumgart, for example, defined the science of medicine as "the entire stockpile of knowledge accumulated about man as a biologic entity. The art of medicine consists in the skillful application of scientific knowledge to a particular person for the maintenance of health or the amelioration of disease. For the individual physician, the meeting place of the science of medicine and the art of medicine is the patient."[66]

Many people believe that the science of medicine has so engulfed physicians and other health professionals that they are no longer interested in the patient as a person. "The patient, it is said, knows how he feels, but does not know what he has, while the doctor knows what the patient has, but does not know how he feels. It is contended that fascination with disease has excluded compassionate regard for the patient who is suffering."[67]

Caring and respect influence patient health outcomes in many ways. Without caring and respect, for instance, communication between patients and providers is often adversely affected. As communication fails, the ability of professionals to effectively diagnose and treat patients tends to diminish sharply.

Consider, for example, the important clinical area of postoperative pain management.[68] Approximately 23.3 million operations were performed in the United States in 1989, and probably more than half of these operations involved some form of *inadequate* postoperative pain management.[68-69] The deeply entrenched "standard" or "routine" procedure of ordering intramuscular injections of some opioid for patients "as needed" ignores the need for effective personalized communication between patients and caregivers. All patients are *not* alike when confronting the prospect or the reality of pain.

Pain has been defined as "a complex, subjective response with several quantifiable features, including intensity, time course, quality, impact, and personal meaning."[70] The communication of pain is a social transaction between caregiver and patient and, according to one source, is the "single most reliable indicator of the existence and intensity of acute pain."[71] Successful assessment and control of postoperative pain depends in part on establishing a positive relationship between health care providers, patients, and, when appropriate, patients' families. Most health professionals agree that adequate postoperative pain management is an ethical obligation, but there are other benefits as well including earlier mobilization, shortened hospital stay, and reduced costs.

The Dimension of Safety

Safety refers to the degree to which the risk of an intervention and the risk in the care environment are reduced for the patient and others, including the health care provider.

The word *safety* is typically applied to organizations' performance in maintaining and improving physical aspects of their environments. Examples include protecting patients, personnel, visitors, and property from fire and the products of combustion;[72] assessing and controlling the clinical and physical risks of fixed and portable equipment used for the diagnosis, treatment, monitoring, and care of patients;[73] and assuring the operational reliability of adequate emergency power systems to provide electricity to designated areas of the organization, such as delivery rooms, operating rooms, and special care units, during interruption of the normal electrical source.[74]

The safety of organizations' physical environments has become an increasingly important topic in recent years as structures age, the demands of modern medical technology steadily increase, and money to invest in meeting minimum safety requirements becomes more scarce. Without adequate attention to the physical environment, organizations place patients, visitors, staff members, and the community at avoidable risk of harm. It is not difficult to imagine scenarios in which equipment that has not been properly maintained fails, leading to undesirable patient health outcomes including death; patients die of smoke inhalation because they cannot escape from a burning building when stairwells are not passable or have not been built; or the community is exposed to radioactive medical waste or used syringes and needles improperly disposed of by health care organizations.

Safety management is a relatively invisible organizational function—that is, it supports direct patient care but often is far removed from patients' and organizational staff members' immediate experience. There is sometimes a temptation to ignore important aspects of safety management in favor of allocating resources to more visible concerns such as purchasing a fixed magnetic resonance imaging machine or some other new and expensive technology.

The word *safety* is sometimes used in its broadest sense, referring not merely to a physically safe environment but also to the performance of physicians and other health professionals working in organizations.[75] In this sense, safety refers to the degree to which patient injury or harm is minimized by minimizing the frequency of inappropriate use of services and by ensuring that practitioners have the knowledge and skills to perform well. Organizational processes such as medical staff credentialing, delineation of clinical privileges, and periodic performance review and reappointment are key processes aimed at achieving these objectives.

From the perspective of patients, purchasers, consumer groups, and others, this second definition of safety is relevant and meaningful. Increasing numbers of people who undergo operations, for example, are asking for objective evidence that the practitioners who are performing operations are competent, experienced, and produce good outcomes.

It is increasingly appreciated that how well organizational systems function is often linked to patient health outcomes. If an organization's blood transfusion system is dysfunctional for any reason, for example, patients who require blood products may experience serious and avoidable complications such as transfusion reactions or death from failure to administer blood products when they are needed. Similarly, if an organization's drug distribution system is faulty, serious medication errors can result.*

Thus, a growing number of patients and purchasers want performance data that not only reflect individual practitioner performance (for example, what is Physician A's rate for performing vaginal deliveries for patients with a previous history of cesarean section?) but also reflect organizational performance in achieving desired outcomes (for example, how many blood transfusion reactions or medication errors occurred in Hospital A last year?)

The Dimension of Timeliness

Timeliness refers to the degree to which the care/intervention is provided to the patient at the time it is most beneficial or necessary.

The timeliness with which organizations meet the needs of patients and other users of organizational services often has a strong influence on health outcomes. The probability that a trauma patient with a gunshot wound to the chest will survive to hospital discharge, that a patient with acute myocardial infarction will benefit from thrombolytic therapy, or that a pediatric patient with acute epiglottitis will receive life-saving airway management is increased when hospital systems (for example, admission, patient assessment, and operative intervention) are functioning in a timely way.

Important organizational services that are not performed in a

---

* The Joint Commission Medication Use Indicator Development Task Force developed the following indicator, which is currently in the beta phase of field testing: "number of reported significant medication errors."

timely manner often result in costly delays. For instance, consider that patients must remain hospitalized additional days because certain services or procedures are not provided when they are needed. Or consider the extra cost associated with keeping all open-heart patients intubated overnight in the intensive care unit because "that's the way it has always been done."

Timeliness issues have been a major focus of the Joint Commission's Trauma Care Task Force for Indicator Development. Some of the indicators this group developed dealt with the timeliness of prehospital emergency medical care, airway management in comatose trauma patients, diagnostic testing for patients with intracranial injury and altered state of consciousness, surgical intervention for adult patients with head injury, surgical intervention for orthopedic injuries, surgical intervention for patients with abdominal injuries, and patient transfer to other institutions.

Multiple Performance Dimensions Help Determine Patient Health Outcomes

The preceding sections focused on the independent importance of each of the dimensions. Equally important is the additive effect of performance regarding several of the dimensions. For example, postoperative wound infections will be reduced if there is a coordinated effort—that is, *continuity* in care—among physicians, pharmacists, nurses, clerks, transporters, and others, to provide the *appropriate* antibiotic in a *timely* and *effective* manner. If any one of these four dimensions is not pursued well, the objective of minimizing postoperative wound infections will not be fully achieved.

Also consider the observation that hospitals that treat a higher volume of patients for certain medical and surgical conditions have better patient health outcomes.[76–79] The achievement of better patient health outcomes in these cases may be due to relatively high levels of, say, performance appropriateness, effectiveness, *and* efficiency.

The dimensions of performance are usually interlinked in relation to processes and outcomes. Efficacy, for example, is often linked to appropriateness because inefficacious procedures are always inappropriate. Timeliness is often linked to efficiency because increasing the level of performance timeliness usually improves efficiency. Effectiveness can be linked to efficiency because a low level of performance effectiveness represents an inefficient use of resources.

The multiple dimensions of performance provide health care organizations with a classification of relevant, well-defined terms useful in designing, measuring, and improving processes and outcomes.

Summary Observations

The important points to be gleaned from this chapter include the following:

1. There are at least nine dimensions along which organizational performance can be measured: appropriateness, availability, continuity, effectiveness, efficacy, efficiency, respect and caring, safety, and timeliness. Each of these performance dimensions are definable, measurable, and improvable.

2. The relative importance of these dimensions is debated and will vary with the situation. An organization's measurement efforts should be sufficiently encompassing and balanced to permit meaningful organizational attention to all of these issues.

3. The dimension of appropriateness refers to the degree to which the care/intervention provided is relevant to the patient's clinical needs, given the current state of knowledge.

4. The dimension of availability refers to the degree to which the appropriate care/intervention is available to meet the needs of the patient served.

5. The dimension of continuity refers to the degree to which the care/intervention for the patient is coordinated among practitioners, between organizations, and across time.

6. The dimension of effectiveness refers to the degree to which the care/intervention is provided in the correct manner, given the current state of knowledge, in order to achieve the desired/projected outcome(s) for the patient.

7. The dimension of efficacy refers to the degree to which the care/intervention used for the patient has been shown to accomplish the desired/projected outcome(s).

8. The dimension of efficiency refers to the ratio of the outcomes (results of care/intervention) for a patient to the resources used to deliver the care.

9. The dimension of respect and caring refers to the degree to

which a patient, or designee, is involved in his or her own care decisions, and that those providing the services do so with sensitivity and respect for his or her needs and expectations and individual differences.

10. The dimension of safety refers to the degree to which the risk of an intervention and the risk in the care environment are reduced for the patient and others, including the health care provider.

11. The dimension of timeliness refers to the degree to which the care/intervention is provided to the patient at the time it is most beneficial or necessary.

12. Multiple performance dimensions usually contribute to patient health outcomes.

References

1. Brook RH, et al. 1989. *Appropriateness of Acute Medical Care for the Elderly: An Analysis of the Literature.* Santa Monica, CA: RAND Corporation.

2. Chassin MR, et al. 1987. Does inappropriate use explain geographic variations in the use of health care services?: A study of three procedures. *JAMA* 258:2533–2537.

3. Chassin MR, et al. 1987. How coronary artery angiography is used. *JAMA* 258:2543–2547.

4. Restuccia JD, et al. 1984. A comparative analysis of appropriateness of hospital use. *Health Aff* 3:130–138.

5. Siu AL, et al. 1988. Use of the hospital in a randomized trial of prepaid care. *JAMA* 259:1343–1346.

6. Siu AL, et al. 1986. Inappropriate use of hospitals in randomized trial of health insurance plans. *New Eng J Med* 315:1259–1266.

7. Winslow CM, et al. 1988. The appropriateness of carotid endarterectomy. *New Eng J Med* 318:721–727.

8. Wells KB, Goldberg G, Brook RH. 1988. Management of patients on psychotropic drugs in primary care clinics. *Med Care* 26:645–657.

9. Merrick NJ, et al. 1986. Use of carotid endarterectomy in five California Veterans Administration Medical Centers. *JAMA* 256:2531–2535.

10. Graboys TB, et al. 1992. Results of a second-opinion trial among patients recommended for coronary angiography. *JAMA* 268:2537–2540.

11. Hillman BJ, et al. 1992. Physicians' utilization and charges for outpatient diagnostic imaging in a Medicare population. *JAMA* 268:2050–2054.

12. Mitchell JM, Scott E. 1992. Physician ownership of physical therapy services: Effects on charges, utilization, profits, and service characteristics. *JAMA* 268:2055–2059.

13. Mitchell JM, Scott E. 1992. New evidence of the prevalence and scope of physician joint ventures. *JAMA* 268:80–84.

14. Waldhoz M, Bogdanich W. 1989. Warm bodies: Doctor-owned labs earn lavish profits in a captive market. *Wall Street J.* March 1:A1, A6.

15. Winslow CM, et al. 1988. The appropriateness of performing coronary artery bypass surgery. *JAMA* 260:505–509.

16. Joint Commission on Accreditation of Healthcare Organizations. 1992. *Trauma, Oncology and Cardiovascular Indicators: Beta Phase Training Manual and Software Users Guide.* Oakbrook Terrace, IL, p 7:44.

17. Willich SN, et al. 1987. High risk subgroups of patients with non-Q wave myocardial infarction based on direction and severity of ST segment deviation. *Am Heart J* 114:1110–1119.

18. Zalenski RJ, et al. 1988. The emergency department ECG and immediately life-threatening complications in initially uncomplicated suspected myocardial ischemia. *Ann Emerg Med* 17:221–226.

19. Lee T, et al. 1991. Rule out acute myocardial infarction. A prospective multicenter validation of a 12-hour strategy for patients at low risk. *New Eng J Med* 324:1239–1246.

20. Ray WA, Griffin MR, Downey W. 1988. Benzodiazepines of long and short elimination half-life and the risk of hip fracture. *JAMA* 262:3303–3307.

21. Woods JH, Katz JL, Winger G. 1988. Use and abuse of benzodiazepines. Issues relevant to prescribing. *JAMA* 260:3476–3480.

22. Joint Commission on Accreditation of Healthcare Organizations. 1992. *Medication Use and Infection Control Indicators: Beta Phase Training Manual and Software Users Guide.* Oakbrook Terrace, IL, p 4:55.

23. Ibid, p 6:54.

24. Atkinson WL, et al. 1990. Transmission of measles in medical settings— United States, 1985–1989. Third International Conference on Nosocomial Infections 1990, p 35.

25. Centers for Disease Control. 1989. General recommendations on immunization, guidelines from the Immunization Practices Advisory Committee. *Ann Intern Med* 111:133–142.

26. Davis RM, et al. 1986. Transmission of measles in medical settings 1980 through 1984. *JAMA* 255:1295–1298.

27. Markowitz LE, et al. 1989. Patterns of transmission in measles outbreaks in the United States, 1985–1986. *N Eng J Med* 320:75–81.

28. Measles—United States, 1989 and first 20 weeks 1990. 1990. *MMWR* 39:353–363.

29. National Coalition for Adult Immunization. 1990. Standards for adult immunization practice. *Am J Hosp Pharm* 47:2348.

30. Sienko DG, et al. 1987. A measles outbreak at university medical settings involving health care providers. *Am J Public Health* 77:1222–1224.

31. *Webster's Deluxe Unabridged Dictionary* 2nd ed. 1979. New York: Simon & Schuster, 1979, p 128.

32. Starr P. 1982. *The Social Transformation of American Medicine.* New York: Basic Books.

33. Stevens R. 1989. *In Sickness and in Wealth: American Hospitals in the Twentieth Century.* New York: Basic Books.

34. Joint Commission on Accreditation of Healthcare Organizations. 1992. Efficiency backrounder. Oakbrook Terrace, IL.

35. Kellermann AL. 1991. Too sick to wait. *JAMA* 266:1123–1124.

36. Baker DW, Stevens CD, Brook RH. 1991. Patients who leave a public hospital without being seen by a physician: Causes and consequences. *JAMA* 266:1085–1090.

37. Bindman AB, et al. 1991. Consequences of queuing for care at a public hospital emergency department. *JAMA* 266:1091–1096.

38. Weissman JS, Gatsonis C, Eptstein AM. 1992. Rates of avoidable hospitalization by insurance status in Massachusetts and Maryland. *JAMA* 268:2388–2394.

39. Buchman AB, Grumbach KV. 1992. America's safety net: The wrong place at the wrong time? *JAMA* 268:2426–2428.

40. Schiff RL, et al. 1986. Transfers to a public hospital: A prospective study of 467 patients. *N Engl J Med* 314:552–557.

41. Himmelstein DU, et al. 1984. Patient transfers: Medical practice as social triage. *Am J Public Health* 74:494–497.

42. Joint Commission on Accreditation of Healthcare Organizations. 1992. *Striving Toward Improvement: Six Hospitals in Search of Quality.* Oakbrook Terrace, IL, pp 116, 147, 218.

43. Ibid, pp 148–153.

44. Ponton TR. 1953. *The Medical Staff in the Hospital.* Chicago: Physician's Record Company, pp 138–139.

45. O'Leary MR, et al. 1988. Physician assessments of practice patterns in emergency department radiograph interpretation. *Ann Emerg Med* 17:1019–1023.

46. O'Leary MR, et al. 1989. Application of clinical indicators in the emergency department. *JAMA* 262:3444–3447.

47. Codman EA. 1934. *The Shoulder: Rupture of the Supraspinatus Tendon and Other Lesions In or About the Subacromial Bursa.* Boston: Thomas Todd Co.

48. Kravitz RL, Rolph JE, McGuigan K. 1991. Malpractice claims data as a quality improvement tool. I. Epidemiology of error in four specialties. *JAMA* 266:2087–2092.

49. Hanft RS. 1983. Monitoring medical technology: Shall technology be regulated: How and by whom? In Gay JR, Sax Jacobs BJ (eds). *The Technology Explosion in Medical Science: Implications for the Health Care Industry and the Public (1981–2001)*. New York: SP Medical & Scientific Books, pp 121–133.

50. Relman AS. 1983. Technology assessment by physicians. In Gay JR, Sax Jacobs BJ (eds). *The Technology Explosion in Medical Science: Implications for the Health Care Industry and the Public (1981–2001)*. New York: SP Medical & Scientific Books, pp 101–109.

51. Morris LC. 1987. Introduction to the Blue Cross and Blue Shield Association guidelines. In Sox HC (ed). *Common Diagnostic Tests: Use and Interpretation*. Philadelphia: American College of Physicians, pp 331–333.

52. Schwartz JS, Ball JF, Moser RN. 1982. Safety, efficacy and effectiveness of clinical practices: A new initiative. *Ann Intern Med* 96:246.

53. American College of Physicians. 1986. *Clinical Efficacy Assessment Project Procedural Manual*. Philadelphia.

54. American College of Physicians. 1988. *Hospital Clinical Privileges: Guidelines for Procedures in Gastroenterology and Nephrology*. Philadelphia.

55. Mushlin AI, Thornbury JR. 1989. Intravenous pyelography: The case against its routine use. *Ann Intern Med* 111:58–70.

56. Nelson D. 1980. *Frederick W. Taylor and the Rise of Scientific Management*. Madison, WI: University of Wisconsin Press.

57. Smiddy H, Naum L. 1979. The evolution of a "science of managing" in America. In Zimet M, Greenwood R (eds). *The Evolving Science of Management: The Collected Papers of Harold Smiddy and Papers by Others in His Honor*. New York: American Management Systems Pub, p 286.

58. Ibid, p 288.

59. Stephenson GW. 1981. The College's role in hospital standardization. *Bull Am Coll Surg* 66:17–29.

60. Schlicke CP. 1973. American surgery's noblest experiment. *Arch Surg* 106(4):379–385.

61. Codman EA: *The Shoulder: Rupture of the Supraspinatus Tendon and Other Lesions In or About the Subacromial Bursa*. Boston: Thomas Todd Co, 1934, p xxii.

62. American Hospital Association. 1991. *Practice Pattern Analysis: A Tool for Continuous Improvement of Patient Care Quality*. Chicago, p 16.

63. Walker AJ. 1990. Results of the Medicare beneficiary and physician focus groups. In Lohr K (ed). *Medicare: A Strategy for Quality Assurance, Volume II: Sources and Methods*. Washington, DC: National Academy Press, pp 45–46.

64. Ibid, p 46.

65. Ibid, p 50.

66. Blumgart H. 1991. Medicine: The art and the science. In Richard R, John S (eds). *On Doctoring.* New York: Simon & Schuster, 1991.

67. Ibid, p 106.

68. US Department of Health and Human Services, Public Health Service, Agency for Health Care Policy and Research. 1992. *Acute Pain Management: Operative or Medical Procedures and Trauma Clinical Practice Guideline,* AHCPR Pub No. 92-0032. Rockville, MD.

69. Peebles RJ, Schneidman DS. 1991. *Socio-Economic Factbook for Surgery, 1991–1992.* Chicago: American College of Surgeons.

70. US Department of Health and Human Services, Public Health Service, Agency for Health Care Policy and Research: *Acute Pain Management: Operative or Medical Procedures and Trauma Clinical Practice Guideline,* AHCPR Pub No. 92-0032. Rockville, MD, Feb 1992, p 7.

71. Ibid, p 11.

72. Joint Commission on Accreditation of Healthcare Organizations. 1991. *Accreditation Manual for Hospitals, Volume I: Standards* 1992 ed. Oakbrook Terrace, IL, p 129.

73. Ibid, p 131.

74. Ibid, p 132.

75. American College of Surgeons. 1985. *Patient Safety Manual* 2nd ed. Chicago, p v.

76. Stone VE, et al. 1992. The relation between hospital experience and mortality for patients with AIDS. *JAMA* 268:2655–2661.

77. Shapiro MR, Greenfield S. 1992. Experience and outcomes in AIDS. *JAMA* 268:2698–2699.

78. Shortell S, LoGerfo J. 1981. Hospital medical staff organization and quality of care: Results for myocardial infarction and appendectomy. *Med Care* 19:1041–1053.

79. Luft HS, Hunt SS, Maerki SC. 1987. The volume-outcome relationship; Practice makes perfect or selective-referral patterns? *Health Serv Res* 22:157–182.

6

Performance Measurement: A Functions-Oriented Approach

There are a variety of approaches to organizing and conducting the process of organizational performance measurement. This chapter focuses on a functions-oriented approach that organizes performance measurement activities along major organizational functions, rather than along structural lines such as departments and offices. A functions-oriented approach to measuring organizational performance is patient centered because it views performance from the perspective of patients who must invariably traverse complex pathways throughout the organization to obtain needed and/or desired services.

Defining a Health Care Organization and Its Functions

Each health care organization has a unique structure that is characterized by a collection of organizational elements, such as departments and offices, and a specific design for their alignment and interaction.[1] Historically, health care organizations have created departments/services to house people with like skills and responsibilities. Thus, accountants reside in the finance department, nurses in the nursing department, and internists in the internal medicine department. While rational, this structure can foster isolation and empire building. One observer likened his hospital, prior to its adoption of a total quality management philosophy and direction, to a "series of fiefdoms connected by a central heating and air conditioning system."[2]

There is sometimes a tendency in such organizations for individual departments to believe that at a practical level the organization exists to support them, rather than the other way around. If an organization does not perform well over time, neither can its departments.[3] There are several incremental approaches to building or rebuilding a common, patient-centered purpose among organizational units including, at the ultimate, cultivation of an organizational culture of continuous improvement in performance. Whatever approach is used, the success with which performance objectives are achieved will depend in large part on the organization's ability to measure and improve its performance of important functions.

What then is a functions-oriented definition of a health care organization? *A health care organization is a system composed of a group of interconnected functions that are carried out to increase the probability that desired patient health outcomes will be achieved.*

What are functions? *A function is a goal-directed group of interconnected processes.*[4] An important function is one believed, on the basis of objective evidence and/or expert consensus, to increase the probability of achieving desired patient health outcomes.

What are processes? As described in Chapter One, *each process is a goal-directed, interrelated series of actions, events, mechanisms, or steps.* An important process is one believed, on the basis of objective evidence and/or expert consensus, to increase the probability of achieving desired patient health outcomes.

The organization that continuously improves performance of its important functions will ultimately achieve improved patient health outcomes. The relationship of a health care organization or system to functions and processes is depicted in Figure 1.

A functions-oriented approach to performance measurement and improvement views the organization's fundamental work as being the provision of good care of patients. The process of taking care of patients is generally the same for every person that enters a health care organization for services. In its simplest form, the process involves a

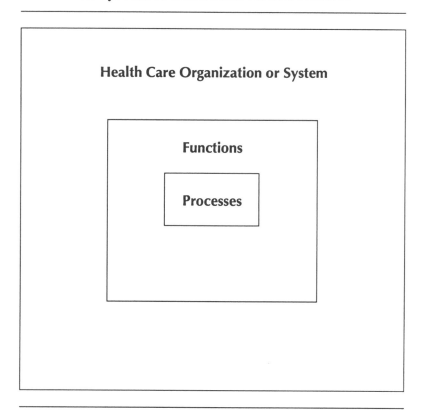

Figure 1

**Relationship of a Health Care Organization
or System to Functions and Processes**

typical patient who enters the organization, is assessed by individuals in the organization, is treated by individuals in the organization, and is discharged from the organization.

Patient Admission to the Organization
↓
Patient Assessment
↓
Patient Treatment
↓
Patient Discharge from the Organization

These four basic activities are important direct patient care functions. Additional patient care functions include nutritional care, patient and family education, and upholding patient rights (see Table 3).[5]

Other important organizational functions support direct patient care functions. These include leadership; human resources management; information management; surveillance, prevention, and control of infection; environmental management; and assessment and improvement of organizational performance (Table 3).[5]

Table 3

Important Organizational Functions and Structures*

Patient Rights

Admission to Setting or Service

Patient Assessment

Nutritional Care

Nonoperative Treatment Selection and Administration

Operative and Other Invasive Procedures

Patient and Family Education

Coordination of Care

Leadership

Human Resources Management

Information Management

Environmental Management

Surveillance, Detection, and Control of Infections

Assessment and Improvement of Organizational
   Performance

Governing Body

Management and Administration

Medical Staff and Nursing

---

*These functions form the basis for the individual chapters of the Joint Commission's *Accreditation Manual for Hospitals,* 1994 edition.

Finally, there are at least four essential structural components of hospitals that exist to support the organization of patient care. These include the governing body, management and administration, the medical staff, and nursing (Table 3).[5]

Important Characteristics of Functions

Functions have a number of important characteristics (see Table 4). *Functions are not uniquely assigned to a specific organizational unit such as an office or a department; rather, more than one unit is usually involved in any given function.* The patient admission function, for example, involves many units. It is a complex process that depends not only on the services performed by the admitting office but also on the performance of other departments and individuals, such as the admitting physician, housekeeping, and nursing services. It is commonplace today for admission to be influenced by medical staff policies, administrative policies, or external requirements.

Functions are performed to achieve desired goals or outcomes, and every function has one or more such goals or outcomes. The goal of the patient assessment function is "to determine treatment through the assessment of the patient's needs in order to achieve desired patient health outcomes."[5] The goal of the leadership function is that "the organization's leaders provide the framework for the planning,

---

Table 4

Characteristics of Organizational Functions

- Involve multiple organizational units such as offices or departments
- Performed to achieve desired goals or outcomes
- Composed of processes
- May be fully, marginally, or only barely visible to patients
- Interlinked throughout the organization
- Support an approach to performance measurement, assessment, and improvement that stresses coordinated, integrated, and efficiently provided services
- Measurable using dimensions of performance

---

direction, coordination, provision, and improvement of health care services which are responsive to the community's and the patient's needs in order to improve patient health outcomes."[5] The goal of the patient and family education function is to "promote recovery, speed return to function, promote good health behaviors, and appropriately involve patients in their care and care decisions in order to improve patient health outcomes."[5]

Ongoing measurement of the level of outcomes achieved as a result of how well functions are performed provides organizations with data and information that are essential for most performance improvement efforts. Important measurable outcomes identified by the Joint Commission Infection Control Indicator Development Task Force for the infection control function include the development of surgical wound infection, postoperative pneumonia, ventilator pneumonia, and endometritis following cesarean section.[6]

All functions are composed of processes. The patient assessment function, for instance, is composed of three important processes: "the gathering of data to assess the needs of the patient; the analysis of these data to create the information necessary to decide the approach to meet patient care or treatment needs; and the making of decisions regarding patient care or treatment based on the analysis of the information."[5] The leadership function is composed of four important processes: "planning for services, directing services, implementing and coordinating services, and improving services."[5]

The potentially large number of processes of which functions are composed form the immediate basis for performance measurement, assessment, and improvement. Consider the infection control function. Several important processes identified by the Joint Commission Infection Control Indicator Development Task Force for ongoing measurement include urinary catheter use in surgical patients; medical abstraction of primary bloodstream infections in patients with a catheter inserted into a major blood vessel, usually through the subclavian or internal jugular vein, or a catheter inserted into the umbilical vein or artery; and immunization of hospital staff for measles.[6] Processes identified by the Joint Commission Medication Use Indicator Development Task Force for ongoing measurement include intravenous preoperative prophylactic antibiotics use and drug level monitoring in patients receiving digoxin, theophylline, phenytoin, or lithium.[6]

Patients will have varying degrees of direct contact with the performance of a function. At one extreme are those patient care functions, such as nutrition and operative and other invasive procedures, that are highly visible to patients and their families. At the other are governance and management and support functions, such as information management and environmental management, that may be invisible to patients and others. Functions such as nonoperative treatment (for instance, medication use) are only partially visible. Each function, however, constitutes a critical element necessary to meet patient needs and foster good patient outcomes.

Functions are invariably interlinked throughout an organization. It is not difficult to imagine how credentialing and privilege delineation processes that fail to consider the organizational resources needed to support a practitioner's new procedure will disrupt the activities of support departments when the procedure is performed. It is also not difficult to imagine how a high level of performance by the organization's information management system can improve the performance of numerous other organizational functions such as surveillance, prevention, and control of infection or measurement, assessment, and improvement of organizational performance.

A functions-oriented approach to performance measurement and improvement stresses the need for individual units of the organization to carry out their activities and responsibilities in a coordinated, integrated, and efficient manner. It enables organizations to emphasize the interlinked and shared responsibilities of individual units in meeting the needs of patients and other users of the organization's services.

Finally, *all functions are measurable using the dimensions of performance* described in Chapter Five. Effectiveness, for instance, is an important dimension of virtually all organizational functions, ranging from operative treatment of patients to organizational leadership. Timeliness is another important dimension that helps to define organizations' performance of functions, ranging from admission of patients to providing information services that meet the needs of users. The appropriateness with which certain functions such as patient assessment, nonoperative treatment, and patient and family education are performed can be measured using performance indicators.

Identifying Measurable Processes and Outcomes Within Individual Functions

A functions-oriented approach to performance measurement requires that an organization identify and select important processes and outcomes within functions. There are several ways in which this can be accomplished.

Flowcharting Functions. Flowcharting is one useful approach to identifying a function's important processes and outcomes. A flowchart is a pictorial summary of the sequence of steps involved in the performance of a function. The Joint Commission is currently developing flowcharts for all of the organizational functions listed in Table 3. Examples of draft flowcharts for the leadership function, the patient and family education function, and the operative and other invasive procedures function are depicted in Figures 2, 3, and 4, respectively.

Flowcharting a function, as opposed to using written or verbal descriptions, has several advantages.[7] It enables people to understand where they fit into a function and how what they do is linked to what others do and the end result of a function. Flowcharts also help to identify particularly important steps and, thereby, highlight them for measurement and monitoring. Flowcharting facilitates detection of problems and opportunities for improvement in a function. Finally, flowcharts provide a record of a function that enables anyone to easily examine, understand, and/or improve the function.

There are several principles governing the technique of flowcharting. First, the people who develop a flowchart should be the "owners" of the function under study—those individuals involved directly in the activity on a day-to-day basis. For example, owners of the operative and other invasive procedures function would include at a minimum physicians (surgeons, anesthetists, emergency physicians, radiologists, pathologists, psychiatrists, intensivists), nurses, pharmacists, information management specialists, managers, clerks, and patients. Exclusion of one or more owners may affect improvement efforts because important input has not been elicited; that input may be key to resolving issues and improving performance and the quality of patient care.

Second, the boundaries of the function under study should be carefully defined. Boundaries make it easier to establish function

Figure 2

Flowchart of the Leadership Function*

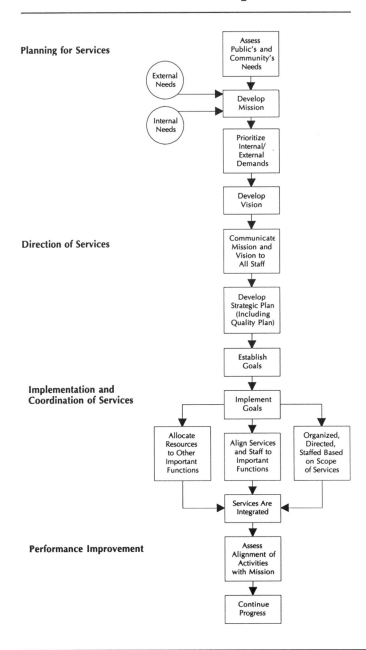

Planning for Services

Assess Public's and Community's Needs

External Needs

Internal Needs

Develop Mission

Prioritize Internal/ External Demands

Develop Vision

Direction of Services

Communicate Mission and Vision to All Staff

Develop Strategic Plan (Including Quality Plan)

Establish Goals

Implementation and Coordination of Services

Implement Goals

Allocate Resources to Other Important Functions

Align Services and Staff to Important Functions

Organized, Directed, Staffed Based on Scope of Services

Services Are Integrated

Performance Improvement

Assess Alignment of Activities with Mission

Continue Progress

*This flowchart was developed by the Joint Commission on Accreditation of Healthcare Organizations Standards Department, 1992. It is currently undergoing testing and is subject to revision.

Figure 3
Flowchart of Patient and Family Education*

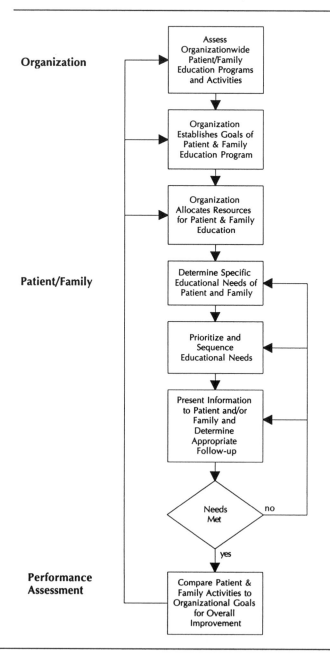

*This flowchart was developed by the Joint Commission on Accreditation of Healthcare Organizations Standards Department. It is currently undergoing testing and is subject to revision.

Figure 4

Flowchart of the Operative and Other Invasive Procedures Function*

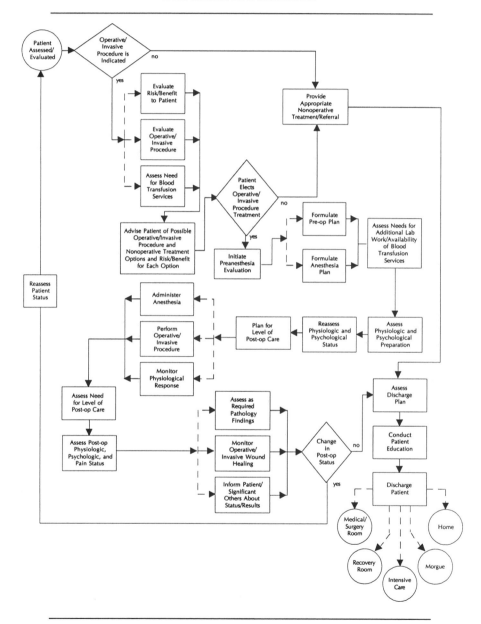

*This flowchart was developed by the Joint Commission on Accreditation of Healthcare Organizations Standards Department. It is currently undergoing testing and is subject to revision.

ownership and highlight the function's interfaces with other functions.[7] For example, the boundaries for a diagnostic imaging function (or subfunction if the function is patient assessment) can be set broadly to include diagnostic imaging services of all types (plain film radiography, computerized axial tomography, magnetic resonance imaging, and other modalities) provided throughout an organization (outpatient department, emergency department, special care units, wards, and other sites). Or the boundaries can be set more narrowly by excluding certain diagnostic imaging services and/or certain sites in which diagnostic imaging services are provided. The boundaries of the trauma care function can be expansive or narrow depending on whether the prehospital, special care unit, rehabilitation, and/or autopsy phases of trauma care are included within the boundaries of the function.

The third principle governing flowcharting is that the key outcomes (both positive and negative) of the function should be identified and measured. Clearly stating the desired goals or outcomes (as well as outcomes to be avoided) of the function helps everyone involved with flowcharting work toward the same goals.

Cause-and-Effect Diagraming of Functions. A second useful approach to identifying the important processes and outcomes that make up a given function is to construct a cause-and-effect diagram of the function. This technique was developed in 1943 by Kaoru Ishikawa and produces what is often called an "Ishikawa chart" or a "fishbone diagram" because a well-constructed diagram takes on the shape of a fish skeleton.

A cause-and-effect diagram helps group members generate and organize theories about the possible causes of a problem or condition (the "effect") and/or enables them to envision causal factors essential to achieving a desired situation. This helps the group plan for data collection so it can pinpoint the actual or most frequently occurring causes. The effect or problem is stated on the right side of the diagram. Group members then brainstorm on the major influences or causes, which are placed as "branches" stemming from the problem or condition. Causes may be subdivided under broad categories such as equipment, policies, and human resources.

The Joint Commission Infection Control Indicator Development

Task Force, for instance, developed the fishbone diagram depicted in Figure 5. The effect, stated on the right side of the diagram, is "reduced nosocomial infection rates," specifically those infections relating to surgical wounds, bloodstream, pneumonia, urinary tract infection (UTI), and employee health. On the left side of the diagram are the major influences or causes leading to reduced nosocomial infection rates. These include surveillance, prevention, and control (the main branches). The cause-and-effect diagram for the health information management function is depicted in Figure 6.

Brainstorming Functions. A third useful approach to identifying the processes and outcomes that make up a function is to brainstorm. This technique has been used at least since the time of the Greeks as a way to elicit a large number of ideas from a group of people in a short period of time. Group members use their collective knowledge and experience to generate ideas and unrestrained thoughts. Brainstorming can be used to develop a list of processes and outcomes that form the immediate basis for measurement as described in Chapter One.

For example, the leadership of a hypothetical hospital may convene a multidisciplinary, multidepartmental group of individuals to brainstorm about the patient assessment function, and, more specifically, about a subfunction, diagnostic imaging. What are the important processes and outcomes that might yield information that could be used to improve that process? Brainstorming would entail each group member listing important processes and outcomes relating to diagnostic imaging. One hypothetical member's list might include the following processes and outcomes:

1. Timely reporting by radiologists of test results to practitioners (a process);
2. Anaphylactoid/anaphylactic reactions to intravenous contrast material (an outcome);
3. Cardiopulmonary arrest of patients while in the radiology suite (an outcome); and
4. Accuracy of radiologists' interpretations of radiographs (an outcome).

Figure 5

Infection Control Function Fishbone Diagram*

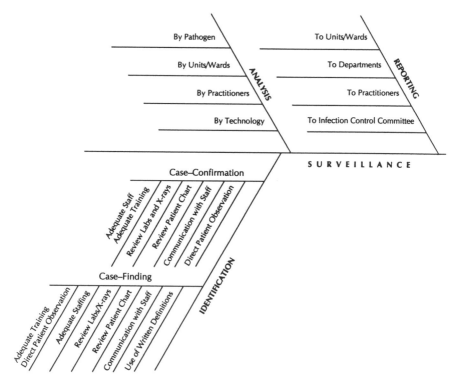

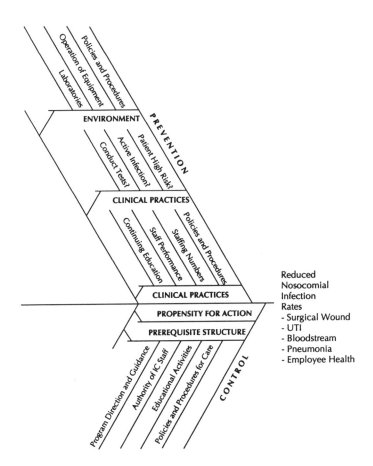

*This fishbone diagram was developed by the Joint Commission Infection Control Indicator Development Task Force

Figure 6
Fishbone Diagram of the Health Information Management Function*

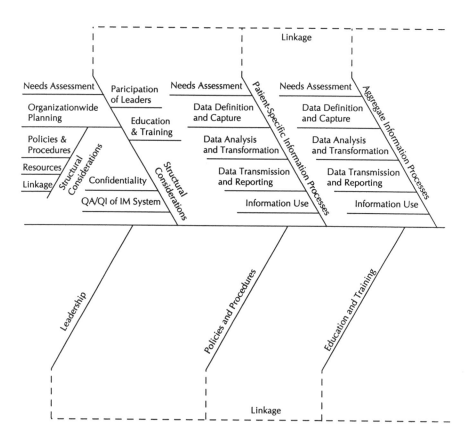

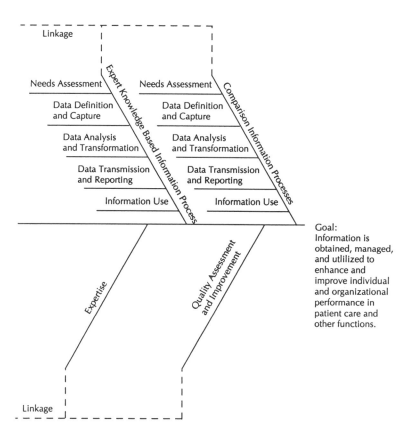

Goal:
Information is obtained, managed, and utlilized to enhance and improve individual and organizational performance in patient care and other functions.

*This fishbone diagram was developed by the Joint Commission Standards Department and is currently undergoing field testing.

Another hypothetical member's list might include the following processes and outcomes:

1. Availability of radiographs for review by practitioners (a process);
2. Missing radiographs (an outcome);
3. Technical quality of radiographs (an outcome); and
4. Appropriate ordering of diagnostic imaging procedures by practitioners (a process).

A third hypothetical member's list might include the following processes and outcomes:

1. Rate of reimbursement for diagnostic imaging procedures, subcategorized by type of procedure (for example, plain film radiography, computerized axial tomography, ultrasonography) (an outcome); and
2. Number of normal (no pathology noted) diagnostic imaging examinations over the total number of diagnostic imaging examinations performed, subcategorized by type of examination (an outcome).

Each group member receives a master list of processes and outcomes that have been suggested for measurement by all of the members of the group. These processes and outcomes are then ranked as to importance by all members of the group. The final ranked list provides the group with its perception of the most important processes and outcomes, and the measurement process can then proceed.

Process and Outcome Variation in Health Care

The functions-oriented approach is well-suited to performance measurement and data analyses. All processes and outcomes display variation.[8–12] Variation is readily displayed by measuring the outputs of a particular process.[13] This variation is unavoidable, yet must be understood, controlled, and reduced to the extent possible. Variation that reflects weak performance frequently leads to waste and loss, such as the occurrence of undesirable patient health outcomes and increased cost of health services.[11]

Consider, for instance, the process of stabilizing and readying for transport trauma patients at the scene of injury.* Scene times in general should be short (20 minutes or less), according to many experts.[14-18] The condition of critically injured patients, such as those with penetrating wounds to the thorax and abdomen, frequently deteriorates over time and the people (surgeons, anesthetists, nurses) and other resources (blood products, diagnostic modalities, operating rooms) needed to definitively assess and treat patients are usually at the hospital, not at the scene of injury or in the ambulance.[14-18] Long scene times—that is, scene times greater than 20 minutes— may result in increased morbidity and mortality and increased costs associated with addressing this morbidity and mortality.[14]

Sources of Variation

There are five main sources of variation in health care and in performance data (see Table 5).[19] *Patient factors* are the wide variety of psychological, economic, social, and physiological variables that relate to the patient and that may or may not be under the control of the health care organization. Examples include severity of illness (the degree or stage of disease prior to treatment); comorbid conditions (disease factors not intrinsic to the primary disease, which may have an impact on patient suitability for, or tolerance of, diagnostic or therapeutic care); and nondisease factors that may have an impact on care, such as age, sex, financial status, and willingness to take risks, but which are not related to illness.

Consider again the trauma care scene time example discussed in the previous section. The patient factors potentially contributing to the variation in length of prehospital scene time described by the Joint Commission Trauma Care Indicator Development Task Force are listed in Table 6.

A second source that may cause variation in health care and in performance data involves *organizational factors*. These factors are usually within the organization's control and influence the nature and effectiveness of care an organization provides. Training nurses in the use of a new intravenous infusion device and educating hospital

---

* The Joint Commission Trauma Care Indicator Development Task Force developed the following indicator, which is currently in the beta phase of field testing: "trauma patients with prehospital emergency medical services (EMS) scene times greater than 20 minutes."

Table 5

Five Sources of Variation
in Health Care Measurement Data[19]

Patient Factors:	the wide variety of psychological, economic, social, and physiological variables that relate to the patient and that may or may not be under the control of a health care organization. Examples of patient factors include severity of illness (factors related to the degree or stage of disease prior to treatment); comorbid conditions (disease factors not intrinsic to the primary disease that may have an impact on patient suitability for, or tolerance of, diagnostic or therapeutic care); other patient factors such as nondisease factors that may have an impact on care (age, sex, financial status, willingness to take risks).
Organizational Factors:	factors within a health care organization's control that influence the underlying average effectiveness of care the hospital provides, such as factors that contribute to the general ability of direct care givers to provide services.
Practitioner Factors:	factors within a health care organization's control that influence the type of assessments and treatments a patient may receive and the effectiveness of those assessments and treatments.
Environmental Factors:	factors, such as nursing home bed availability and payer reimbursement policies, with which a health care organization must cope even though the factors are outside of the health care organization's control.
Chance Variation:	random variation in the patient, organization, practitioner, and/or environmental factors.

Table 6

Potential Underlying Factors Contributing to Variation in Prehospital Scene Times for Trauma Patients*

Patient Factors:
1. Severity of illness
   a. difficult airway control
   b. multiple fractures
   c. traumatic cardiac arrest
2. Comorbid conditions
   a. disruptive patients
   b. difficult intravenous access
3. Other patient factors
   a. problematic extrication
   b. multiple trauma patients
   c. scene control problems
   d. delayed ambulance arrival
   e. patient communication problems

Organizational Factors:
1. Adequacy and appropriateness of standing medical orders
2. Nature and quality of training of personnel
3. Equipment functioning
4. Appropriateness and sufficiency of dispatch of personnel to scene
5. Adequacy of medical control
6. Adequacy of supplies

Practitioner Factors:
1. Adequacy of training or experience of prehospital personnel
2. Appropriateness of techniques used by prehospital personnel
3. Health of health care practitioners
4. Compliance of prehospital personnel in following protocols
5. Contact or maintenance of contact with hospital-based medical personnel

* Developed by the Joint Commission Trauma Care Indicator Development Task Force. The following indicator is in the beta phase of field testing: "trauma patients with prehospital emergency medical services (EMS) scene greater than 20 minutes."

staff about universal infection control procedures are examples of organizational factors that can contribute to the general ability of practitioners to provide effective and safe services. Organizational factors are often the object of thorough performance measurement, assessment, and improvement processes. The organizational factors potentially influencing variation in length of prehospital scene time for trauma patients are listed in Table 6.

Practitioner factors are a third source that may cause variation in health care and performance data. They are individual practitioner-related factors usually within the health care organization's control which influence the type of assessments and treatments a patient may receive and the effectiveness of those assessments and treatments. Adequate training and experience, for instance, is an important practitioner factor that can influence the type of assessment and treatment a patient receives. The practitioner factors potentially influencing variation in length of prehospital scene time for trauma patients are listed in Table 6.

A fourth source of variation in health care measurement data involves *chance or random variation* (often called "error" by statisticians) in patient, organization, and/or practitioner factors.

Environmental factors, a fifth potential source of variation in health care and performance data, include payer reimbursement policies, availability of health care resources in the community (for example, nursing home beds), and availability of health care practitioners (for example, primary care physicians, nurses, respiratory therapists). Environmental factors may strongly affect the nature of the quality of care provided by an organization. While not directly controllable by the organization, they are factors with which many organizations must constantly cope.

Two Types of Variation: Common and Special

There are two types of variation.[8-12] The first type—sometimes called *common cause* variation, endogenous cause variation, or systemic cause variation—is always present and is part of the variation inherent in all processes. Common causes of variation are endogenous to a system and are not disturbances (they *are* the system) and can be removed or eliminated only by making basic changes in the system. Often these changes are highly desirable and constitute the substrate of continuous improvement projects and efforts.

The origins of common cause variation can usually be traced to an element of the system that the organization can correct and improve. Some sources of common cause variation include design of a system, choice of equipment, and preventive maintenance of equipment. Dr WE Deming cites additional examples, including worn or outdated equipment; inadequate instruction and/or supervision of employees; poor lighting; failure to provide workers with statistical information to help them improve performance and reduce variation; and unpleasant working conditions.[20] In the prehospital scene time example discussed previously, potential sources of common cause variation include all of the items listed under organizational factors (see Table 6).

Organizational management frequently holds employees responsible for common cause problems when the problems have been actually built into the process. Management that is concerned with the amount of common cause variation in a process must act to reduce it. Some experts estimate that common variation causes about 85% of the problems in a process while 15% are caused by special variation, described below.[11]

Consider, for example, a hospital's system for providing treatment for severely ill patients in one of the hospital's special care units. Some of these patients will die because of the severity of their primary illness and/or other patient-based factors such as age. Although the special care unit mortality rate attributable to patient-based factors will vary somewhat over time, the amplitude of the variation is usually small and within predictable limits. A certain number of deaths occur not because of an inadequate system for providing intensive care; rather, these deaths occur because of the nature of the patients in the system.

Or consider an organization's system for interpreting plain film radiographs—a process that contributes to the patient assessment function. There is an interradiologist disagreement rate of up to 10%, suggesting that there is an irreducible minimum of variant performance even among those individuals considered most qualified by training and experience to interpret radiographs.[21-24] A certain disagreement rate occurs *not* because the system for interpreting radiographs is necessarily inadequate. Rather, disagreements occur because well-trained and experienced individuals nevertheless will have a small but measurable number of differences. The interradiologist disagreement rate will vary somewhat over time; its amplitude, however, will usually remain relatively stable and within predictable limits over time.

A second type of variation—sometimes called *special cause* variation, assignable cause variation, attributable cause variation, exogenous cause variation, or extrasystemic cause variation—is *not inherently* present in the system itself. Rather, it arises from causes that are not part of the system as designed. Special cause variation is intermittent and indicates that a process is unstable.[11]

When special causes are operating within a system or process, the output of that system or process is impossible to predict or control. The process or system is "in a state of chaos"—that is, "it is producing some nonconforming product [or service] and it is not in a state of statistical control. There is no way to know or predict the percentage of nonconforming products [or patient health outcomes] that the process will generate."[11] Ideally, once detected, special causes of variation that result in undesirable outcomes can and should be eliminated by an organization, leaving a process with only common causes of variation.

Extrasystemic causes tend to cluster by person, place, and time. Consider, for example, that there is a sharp acceleration of deaths in a hospital unit. As soon as this pattern is identified, immediate in-depth investigation becomes imperative because an unusual number of deaths in a given time period suggests that specific and identifiable causes may exist that can and must be eliminated. In two hospitals, for example, epidemics of deaths were traced to practitioners who apparently were administering lethal doses of substances such as digoxin and potassium to patients.[25-26] The culpable individuals here are the special causes of observed variation in mortality because they clearly were not part of the intended system of care. Removal of the practitioners permits the care systems to return to their relatively low, relatively predictable mortality rate.

Suppose that an organization's interrater disagreement rate for interpretation of radiographs suddenly jumps to 30% from its usual baseline rate of between 0% and 10%. This suggests that a specific and identifiable cause, such as a compromised practitioner or technician or a change in the film development process, may exist that can and should be removed to return the disagreement rate to its baseline rate of variation.

Occasionally, extrasystemic causes can result in better outcomes. When identified, these desirable special causes should be incorporated into the conventional system so that better outcomes do recur.

How can one make a distinction between common and special cause variation? Control charts are important statistical tools that make this distinction possible.[11] Control charts and other data analysis tools are described in detail elsewhere.[19, 27–30]

Summary Observations

The concept of functions is key to understanding organizational performance measurement. The important ideas in this chapter include the following:

1. A health care organization is a system composed of a group of interconnected functions that are carried out to increase the probability that desired patient health outcomes will be achieved.

2. A function is a goal-directed set of interconnected processes. Essential organization functions include those that involve direct patient care, such as patient assessment and patient treatment, and those that support direct patient care, such as leadership and human resources management. Processes of which functions are composed form the immediate basis for performance measurement, assessment, and improvement.

3. Functions have many important characteristics. An individual function is not uniquely assigned to a specific organizational unit such as a department; rather, more than one unit is usually involved in any given function. A function is made up of processes and is goal directed. From the patient's perspective, all functions lie along a continuum ranging from functions that are visible to the patient, such as direct patient care functions, to functions with relatively low visibility to the patient, such as the environmental management function. Functions are invariably interlinked. A functions-oriented approach to performance measurement and improvement stresses the need for individual units of the organization to carry out their activities and responsibilities in a coordinated, integrated, and efficient manner. A functions-oriented approach to performance measurement and improvement is patient centered. Performance of functions is measurable using dimensions of performance such as effectiveness and appropriateness.

4. Flowcharting, cause-and-effect diagraming, and brainstorming are three useful techniques to identify important processes and outcomes that comprise functions for measurement and improvement purposes.

5. Processes and outcomes in health care always display variation.

6. There are five potential sources of variation: patient based, organization based, practitioner based, environment based, and chance.

7. There are two types of variation: common cause variation and special cause variation. These two types of variation can be effectively distinguished with control charts.

References

1. Joint Commission on Accreditation of Healthcare Organizations. 1990. *Primer on Indicator Development and Application.* Oakbrook Terrace, IL, pp 23–26.

2. Joint Commission on Accreditation of Healthcare Organizations. 1992. *Striving Toward Improvement: Six Hospitals in Search of Quality.* Oakbrook Terrace, IL, p 46.

3. O'Leary DS, O'Leary MR. 1992. From quality assurance to quality improvement: The Joint Commission on Accreditation of Healthcare Organizations and emergency care. *Emergency Clinics of North America* 10:477–492.

4. Joint Commission on Accreditation of Healthcare Organizations. 1990. *Primer on Indicator Development and Application.* Oakbrook Terrace, IL, p 111.

5. Joint Commission proposed standards for the 1994 *Accreditation Manual for Hospitals* as of November 6, 1992.

6. Joint Commission on Accreditation of Healthcare Organizations. 1992. *Medication Use and Infection Control Indicators: Beta Phase Training Manual and Software User's Guide.* Oakbrook Terrace, IL.

7. Gitlow H, et al. 1989. *Tools and Methods for the Improvement of Quality.* Homewood, IL: Irwin, p 46.

8. Shewhart WA. 1925. The application of statistics as an aid in maintaining quality of a manufactured product. *J Am Stat Assoc* 20:546–548.

9. Deming WE. 1986. *Out of the Crisis.* Cambridge, MA: Massachusetts Institute of Technology, Center for Advanced Engineering Study.

10. Juran JM. 1964. *Managerial Breakthrough.* New York: McGraw-Hill International Book Co.

11. Gitlow H, et al. 1989. *Tools and Methods for the Improvement of Quality.* Homewood, IL: Irwin, pp 162–164.

12. Kritchevsky SB, Simmons BP. 1991. Continuous quality improvement: Concepts and applications for physician care. *JAMA* 266:1817–1823.

13. Goal/QPC. 1988. *The Memory Jogger* 2nd ed. Methuen, MA, p 85.

14. Ninth Annual Meeting of the Association for Health Services Research and the Foundation for Health Services Research: Joint Commission's Trauma Indicator Development Form, TR-1: Trauma patients with prehospital emergency medical scene times greater than 20 minutes. 1992. In *Methods Workshop: The Joint Commission Indicator Monitoring System: Quality Improvement in Action.* Chicago, June 7–9, pp 63–67.

15. American College of Surgeons, Committee on Trauma. 1987. Hospital and prehospital resources for optimal care of the injured patient. *Bull of the ACS;* Appendix G; No. 2.

16. Gervin AS, Fischer RP. 1982. The importance of prompt transport and salvage of patients with penetrating heart wounds. *J Trauma* 22:443–448.

17. Pons PT, et al. 1985. Prehospital advanced trauma life support for critical penetrating wounds to the thorax and abdomen. *J Trauma* 25:828–832.

18. Cwinn AA, et al. 1987. Prehospital advanced life support for critical blunt trauma victims. *Ann Emerg Med* 16:399–403.

19. Joint Commission on Accreditation of Healthcare Organizations. 1992. *Beta II Feedback Report; Trauma Indicators, 1992, Quarters I & II.* Oakbrook Terrace, IL, pp 9–29.

20. Deming WE. 1982. *Quality, Productivity and Competitive Position.* Cambridge, MA: Massachusetts Institute of Technology, Center for Advanced Engineering Study, p 116.

21. Herman PG, Hessel SJ. 1975. Accuracy and its relationship to experience in the interpretation of chest radiographs. *Invest Radiol* 10:62–67.

22. Berlin L. 1977. Does the "missed" radiographic diagnosis constitute malpractice? *Radiology* 123:523–536.

23. Swennsson RG, Hessel SJ, Herman PG. 1977. Omissions in radiology: Faulty search or stringent reporting criteria? *Radiology* 123:563–567.

24. Rhea FT, Potsaid MS, DeLuca SA. 1979. Errors of interpretation as elicited by a quality audit of an emergency radiology facility. *Radiology* 132:277–280.

25. Buehler JW, et al. 1985. Unexplained deaths in a children's hospital: An epidemiologic assessment. *N Eng J Med* 313:211–216.

26. Sacks JJ, Stroup DR, Will ML. 1988. A nurse-associated epidemic of cardiac arrests in an intensive care unit. *JAMA* 259:689–695.

27. Gitlow H, et al. 1989. *Tools and Methods for the Improvement of Quality.* Homewood, IL: Irwin, pp 164–213.

28. Joint Commission on Accreditation of Healthcare Organizations. 1991. *Development and Application of Indicators in Emergency Care.* Oakbrook Terrace, IL, pp 47–74.

29. Joint Commission on Accreditation of Healthcare Organizations. 1991. *Development and Application of Indicators for Continuous Improvement in Surgical and Anesthesia Care.* Oakbrook Terrace, IL, pp 53–76.

30. Joint Commission on Accreditation of Healthcare Organizations. 1992. *Development and Application of Indicators for Continuous Improvement in Perinatal Care.* Oakbrook Terrace, IL, pp 45–66.

7

How a Performance Measurement System Works

A performance measurement system is composed of a sequence of three basic steps: establishment of units of measure, development and validation of instruments capable of reliably quantifying the units of measure, and use of the instruments to produce measurement data for subsequent analysis and use in the performance improvement process (see Table 7).[1] Each of these measurement steps must be performed well to provide the information needed for effective improvement. The degree, for example, that collected data are accurate and complete will have a substantive impact on the degree to which the data can or will be trusted by potential users of the data.

The First Step: Establishing Units of Measure

The first step in a performance measurement system is establishment of units of measure. A unit of measure, as described in detail in Chapter One, is a defined amount of an attribute of a person, an activity, or a thing (such as an object, an event, or a phenomenon). Classic units of measure include, for instance, a meter (an amount of length), a quart (an amount of volume), and a Celsius degree (an amount of heat). Length, volume, and heat are attributes of things that scaled units of measure quantify.

Table 7

Three Steps of a Performance Measurement System

- •Step 1   Establish units of measure.
- •Step 2   Develop instruments capable of quantifying the units of measure.
- •Step 3   Use instruments to produce measurement data for subsequent analysis and use in the performance improvement process.

In measuring performance in health care, common units of measure relate to the patient, a procedure, or a condition. Timeliness, appropriateness, effectiveness, and the other dimensions of performance described in Chapter Five are common attributes for which health care organizations develop such units of measure.

The timeliness with which a diagnostic modality is employed is a dimension, for instance, that can be measured by an indicator such as "trauma patients with a diagnosis of intracranial injury and altered state of consciousness on emergency department arrival who receive an initial head computerized tomography scan less than two hours after emergency department arrival."* In this example, the unit of measure is the trauma patient with a diagnosis of intracranial injury and altered state of consciousness on emergency department arrival who receives initial head computerized tomography scan less than two hours after emergency department arrival. The total number of such patients is compared to the overall number of trauma patients with diagnosis of intracranial injury and altered state of consciousness upon arrival to the emergency department seen by the hospital within an identified period (for example, six months). This comparison of numbers can lead to a rate, or proportion, that tells the hospital what percentage of head-trauma patients are receiving timely diagnostic testing for their condition.

---

* The Joint Commission Trauma Care Indicator Development Task Force developed the following analogous indicator, which is currently in the beta phase of field testing: "trauma patients with diagnosis of intracranial injury and altered state of consciousness upon emergency department arrival receiving initial head computerized tomography scan greater than two hours after emergency department arrival."

Establishment of units of measure is a challenge to some health care organizations for the same set of reasons that performance measurement in general is challenging (see Chapter Three). These reasons include health care provider concerns about disclosure of performance data and information, perceived threats to traditional professional autonomy, negative attitudes developed during the quality assurance era, and severe capital and other resource constraints experienced by increasing numbers of health care organizations.

There are several other reasons why health care organizations may grapple with development of units of measure. Virtually all important organizational performance attributes have been formerly judged by human perception, not through the development and application of precise measurement units.[2] People are accustomed to communicating their perception of performance level with phrases such as "high-quality hospital," "good nurse," "competent doctor," "effective administrator," and "efficient emergency services system" or "best oncology services." Development of units of measure that quantify these human judgments requires discipline, thoughtfulness, education, and willingness to change.

Second, variation in opinion among organizations and professionals both inside and outside of the health care sector may exist as to which units of measure are valid measures of organizational performance. No one can really know for sure because experience with measuring organizational and professional performance of an everyday nature has been, until recently, extremely limited.

Third, many health care organizations are structured in ways that may inhibit the collaboration, coordination, and communication among departments and offices that are essential to successful performance measurement and improvement strategies. The barriers between and among departments and disciplines must be crossed to develop units of measure that, when used, can lead to improvement. Fourth, the public demand for performance data and information places health care organizations under pressure to produce these data within a relatively short time frame.

A functions-oriented approach to performance measurement (see Chapter Six) can improve the ability of organizations to establish valid units of measure in a more efficient time frame. First, a functions-oriented approach requires a multidepartmental, multidisciplinary team effort in almost all organizational improvement activities beginning with the conceptualization of units of measure. A functions-oriented approach views patient care from the perspective of patients, thus prompting measurement that tracks care across disciplines and departments.

As experienced by the patient, admission involves a series of steps that are critical to efficient entry into the organization and timely access to needed services. Measurement of the admissions function must relate to both the key steps in the multidepartmental, multidisciplinary effort and to the outcomes of the processes. Flow-charting the admissions function can enable an organization to gather representatives from all relevant departments and disciplines in a team that efficiently conceptualizes and establishes valid units of measure.

A functions-oriented approach to performance measurement can also foster cooperative efforts among the individuals involved in a function—that is, the individuals with the breadth of knowledge and experience necessary to develop valid units of measure. In addition to looking internally for such expertise, most organizations will benefit from learning how other organizations carry out important functions. Finally, a functions-oriented approach is ideal for brainstorming, a technique used to elicit a large number of ideas from a group of people in a short period of time.[3]

The Second Step: Developing Measurement Instruments

The second step in performance measurement is to develop an instrument that is calibrated in terms of the unit of measure. The instrument used in many performance measurement systems, including the Joint Commission's indicator monitoring system described later, is called an *indicator* (Table 8, Figure 7).[4] There are two major types of indicators with which the Joint Commission has had considerable experience: aggregate data indicators and sentinel event indicators.

Aggregate Data Indicators

The first major type of performance measure is an aggregate data indicator (Table 8, Figure 7). An *aggregate data indicator* quantifies a process or an outcome related to many cases, as opposed to isolated

Table 8
Important Indicator Definitions

Aggregate data indicator: A performance measure based on collection and aggregation of data about many events or phenomena. The events or phenomena may be desirable or undesirable, and the data may be reported as a continuous variable or as a discrete variable (or rate).

Continuous variable indicator: An aggregate data indicator in which the value of each measurement can fall anywhere along a continuous scale (for example, the precise weight in pounds of an individual receiving total parenteral nutrition).

Rate-based (or discrete variable) indicator: An aggregate data indicator in which the value of each measurement is expressed as a proportion or as a ratio. In a proportion, the numerator is expressed as a subset of the denominator (for example, patients with cesarean section over all patients who deliver). In a ratio, the numerator and denominator measure different phenomena (for example, the number of patients with central lines who develop infections over central line days).

Sentinel event indicator: A performance measure that identifies an individual event or phenomenon that always triggers further analysis and investigation and that usually occurs infrequently and is undesirable in nature.

cases, as in a sentinel event indicator (see the following section). Aggregate data indicators can be developed to measure either a discrete variable or a continuous variable.

A *discrete variable* is a measurement that is limited to discrete options (for example, yes *or* no *or* unknown; less than or equal to 20 minutes *or* greater than 20 minutes). Thus, an aggregate indicator that measures a discrete variable classifies an event as to whether it falls into one discrete category or another, as in, the event occurs *or* does not occur, or the event takes more than one hour *or* less than one hour.

An aggregate data indicator that measures a discrete variable is called a *rate-based indicator* or a *discrete variable indicator*. Clinical examples include whether prehospital scene time for a trauma patient

Figure 7

Relationship of Aggregate Data, Sentinel Event, Continuous Variable, and Discrete Variable (Rate-Based) Indicators

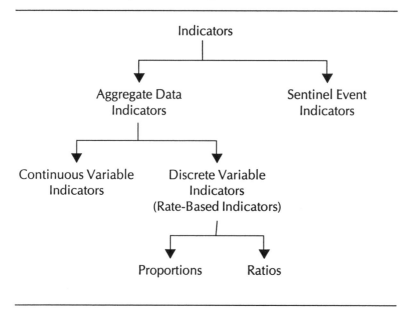

is greater than 20 minutes *or* less than or equal to 20 minutes;* whether a neonate is discharged with *or* without a diagnosis of significant birth trauma;† whether a client receiving total parenteral nutrition and/or enteral therapy is achieving or maintaining, *or* not achieving or maintaining, desired weight;‡ and whether operative

---

* The Joint Commission Trauma Care Indicator Development Task Force developed the following indicator, which is currently in the beta phase of field testing: "trauma patients with prehospital emergency medical services scene time greater than 20 minutes."

† The Joint Commission Obstetrical Care Indicator Development Task Force developed the following indicator, which is currently in the beta phase of field testing: "neonates with a discharge diagnosis of significant birth trauma."

‡ The Joint Commission Home Infusion Therapy Indicator Development Task Force developed the following indicator, which is currently in the beta phase of field testing: "clients receiving total parenteral nutrition and/or enteral therapy who are achieving or maintaining desired weight."

reports of patients with resection of primary colorectal cancer include, *or* do not include, location of primary tumor, local extent of disease, extent of resection, and assessment of residual abdominal disease.* Data expressed by indicators that are founded on classifying items, such as events or phenomena, into at least two categories are called *discrete variable data.*

A *continuous variable* is a measurement that can fall anywhere along a continuous scale (for example, precise number of minutes for response to a call). An aggregate data indicator that measures a continuous variable is called a *continuous variable indicator.* Clinical examples include indicators that measure the precise weight of patients receiving total parenteral nutrition and/or enteral therapy; the precise number of minutes spent at the prehospital emergency medical services scene by trauma patients; or the precise number of days taken from the time of patient referral (including self-referral) to initiation of treatment at a mental health care facility.

The actual values for each continuous variable (the weight, in pounds, of patients receiving total parenteral nutrition; the time, in minutes, spent at the prehospital scene; the time, in days, between patient referral and initiation of treatment at a mental health care facility) are recorded, and through the use of statistical process control techniques (for example, x-bar and R charts), the process or outcome is monitored. Actions are taken either to intentionally eliminate special causes of variation (see Chapter Six), or to make incremental improvements. Data that are expressed by indicators founded on measuring a characteristic, such as time or weight, of a process or an outcome are called *continuous variable data.*[5]

Consider the indicator that quantifies the days taken from the time of patient referral (including self-referral) to initiation of treatment at a mental health care facility. This indicator can be changed from measuring a continuous variable to measuring a discrete variable simply by imposing an arbitrary cutoff so that it detects only those patients seen, for instance, *more than two weeks* from initial referral.

---

* The Joint Commission Oncology Care Indicator Development Task Force developed the following indicator, which is currently in the beta phase of field testing: "patients with primary colorectal cancer whose operative reports include location of primary tumor, local extent of disease, extent of resection, and assessment of residual abdominal disease."

Similarly, the indicator, "trauma patients with prehospital emergency medical services scene times greater than 20 minutes"* can be modified to measure a continuous variable: "prehospital emergency medical services scene time (in minutes)."

When using an aggregate data indicator composed of discrete variables, the indicator—a rate-based (or discrete variable) indicator—is usually expressed as a rate, based on the population at risk. A rate-based indicator may express data either as a proportion or ratio. A *proportion* defines the numerator as a subset of the denominator—for example, the number of mothers with primary cesarean sections and failure to progress divided by the number of mothers with primary cesarean sections or:

$$\frac{\text{Number of mothers with primary cesarean sections and failure to progress}}{\text{Number of mothers with primary cesarean sections}^\dagger}.$$

A *ratio* describes the population at risk in terms other than numbers of patients. For example, the indicator, "inpatients with a central or umbilical line who develop primary bloodstream infections" utilizes a denominator of "central or umbilical line days," leading to a calculated ratio of patients with primary bloodstream infections divided by central or umbilical line days or:

$$\frac{\text{Inpatients with a central or umbilical line who develop primary bloodstream infections}}{\text{Central or umbilical line days}^\ddagger}.$$

---

* The Joint Commission Trauma Care Indicator Development Task Force developed the following indicator, which is currently in the beta phase of field testing: "trauma patients with prehospital emergency medical services scene time greater than 20 minutes."

† The Joint Commission Obstetrical Care Indicator Development Task Force developed the following indicator, which is currently in the beta phase of field testing: "patients with primary cesarean section for failure to progress."

‡ The Joint Commission Infection Control Indicator Development Task Force developed this indicator, which is currently in the beta phase of field testing.

Which type of indicator is more useful—a continuous variable indicator or a discrete variable indicator? The general consensus is that indicators measuring continuous variables and, thereby, generating continuous variable data, are more powerful than those measures built on discrete data. This is because data they generate contain more information, and additional statistical techniques can be used to assess the data.[5-6]

Consider again the time taken between patient referral and initiation of treatment at a mental health care facility. When an arbitrary cutoff point of two weeks is imposed, as described, the indicator is less useful for monitoring and improving underlying process(es) *if few patients require more than two weeks to receive treatment.* When the indicator is changed to quantify a continuous variable (the precise number of days), it can be useful to know whether individual patients take one week or one month to receive treatment. This usefulness derives from the capacity of the measurement to detect aggregated incremental changes in responses to modifications to the underlying process(es).

When the underlying variables are continuous variables, a decision to convert them into discrete variables for performance measures (for example, recording prehospital emergency medical services scene times of either less than or equal to 20 minutes *or* greater than 20 minutes, rather than the actual time) may relate to desired efficiency in measuring and recording the data or the use to which the performance measure is to be put.

Statistical process control techniques are commonly used by organizations to monitor events or phenomena. However, in order to permit internal or external comparisons, indicator data must be expressed in a form that incorporates a denominator. It is the denominator that permits a meaningful comparison.

By their nature, discrete variable data for an indicator include a denominator. But for continuous variable data, additional calculations are required. These would usually define the characteristics of the population of the event or phenomenon in terms of a mean and a standard deviation. These calculations use denominators (for example, the number of patients for which the continuous variable of prehospital emergency medical services scene time was measured) to characterize the performance (for example, the average scene time each month). Thus for *comparative* purposes, discrete variable data are expressed as "rates" (either as ratios or proportions), while continuous variable indicator data are usually expressed as means (and standard deviations).

Sentinel Event Indicators

A *sentinel event indicator* identifies an individual event or phenomenon that always triggers further analysis and investigation each time the event or phenomenon occurs. As described in detail elsewhere, the event or phenomenon measured by a sentinel event indicator is usually undesirable but may be desirable, and it usually occurs infrequently but in some instances may occur frequently.[4]

When data collected for indicator calculations are analyzed as separate cases, these individual cases are labeled as sentinel events. Examples of sentinel event indicators include "patients with unplanned respiratory arrest during or within one postprocedure day involving anesthesia administration"* and maternal death. Each case identified by these indicators is analyzed as a *sentinel event*.

Sentinel event indicators are generally viewed as being of limited value because they represent the extremes of performance measurement. In this regard, their most practical applications relate to risk management activities. Even then, analysis and investigation of a sentinel event may prove to be inconclusive.

Despite their low frequency, there may be value in aggregating sentinel events in a fashion that would resemble a discrete variable indicator. Such aggregation may occasionally be possible in an individual organization but more commonly will be feasible in a large performance database. When sentinel events of the same or similar nature are aggregated, they may prove to be a richer source of information for analysis than the individual events alone.

An alternative approach to the use of sentinel event indicators is to group related indicators into a single numerator (for example, those that measure the number of patients with acute myocardial infarction, patients with stroke, and patients with respiratory arrest during the perioperative period). In this discrete variable indicator,

---

* The Joint Commission Anesthesia Care Indicator Development Task Force developed this indicator, which is currently in the beta phase of field testing.

the rough denominator might be all anesthesia cases. Again, the purpose of attempting to create such artificial discrete variable indicators is to provide a potentially enhanced base of information for analysis.

Important Characteristics of Aggregate Data Indicators

An aggregate data indicator is a versatile instrument with several important characteristics (see Table 9). *The first important characteristic is that it usually measures an event or a phenomenon that is expected to occur with some level of frequency.* Consider the rate-based indicator dealing with indwelling urinary catheter use in surgical patients.* A certain proportion of patients undergoing selected surgical operations will require urinary catheters for greater than 48 hours postoperatively for appropriate reasons such as ongoing urinary retention or state of unconsciousness.

There are situations, however, in which the use of indwelling urinary catheters is inappropriate. These situations include, for instance, ordering indwelling urinary catheters out of habit or for staff members' convenience, and inertia in ordering or actually removing catheters in a timely matter.[7–13] Indicator data showing either a high or a significantly increased use of catheters should prompt evaluation.

The Joint Commission is currently conducting beta testing of indicators developed by its indicator development task forces. One important objective of the beta testing phase of indicator development is to assess the quality of the data that are being transmitted to the Joint Commission from participating beta test site hospitals. Early data are showing which indicator rates are relatively high—meaning that the event or phenomenon measured by the indicator is occurring with some level of frequency—and which indicator rates are not.

Examples of relatively high rates from individual hypothetical hospitals are provided in following paragraphs with the important

---

*The Joint Commission Infection Control Indicator Development Task Force developed the following indicator, which is currently in the beta phase of field testing: "selected surgical procedures on inpatients who are catheterized during the perioperative period."

Table 9

Characteristics of Aggregate Data Indicators

- Measure events or phenomena that are expected to occur with some level of frequency.

- Express data about either a process or an outcome.

- Provide organizations with an early warning of performance areas requiring attention.

- Express data about occurrences that are either desirable or undesirable.

- Express data that guide organizations in improving their norms of performance instead of focusing exclusively on censoring or eliminating individual outliers.

---

caveat that a variety of factors may undermine the reliability and accuracy of these test data. These factors include indicator data element definitional ambiguities; indicator software problems; hospital downloading programs that fail to match specifications; inadequate test site knowledge about how to use the software; inadequate test site knowledge about the indicators; variation in test site ICD-9-CM coding practices; variation in the quality and quantity of physician-provided information; variation in the quality and quantity of patient-provided information; variation in the test site's commitment to beta testing; variation in the quantity of hospitals' resources available for beta testing; and variation in hospital practices, policies, and procedures.[14]

Obstetrical examples in individual hypothetical hospitals include the average or mean indicator occurrence rate of approximately 47% for patients who receive primary cesarean section for failure to progress (Figure 8);[15,] * approximately 7% for patients with excessive

---

* The Joint Commission Obstetrical Care Indicator Development Task Force developed the following indicator, which is currently in the beta phase of field testing: "patients with primary cesarean section for failure to progress."

maternal blood loss (Figure 9);[16,*] and approximately 81% for patients with successful vaginal birth after previous cesarean section (Figure 10).[17,†]

Nonobstetrical examples in individual hypothetical hospitals include the mean indicator occurrence rate of approximately 66% for patients with resections of primary colorectal cancer whose preoperative evaluation by a managing physician includes examination of the entire colon, liver function tests, chest x-ray, and carcinoembryonic antigen (CEA) levels (Figure 11);[18,‡] approximately 38% for prehospital emergency medical services (EMS) scene times (for trauma patients) of greater than 20 minutes (Figure 12)[19,§]; and approximately 82% for patients with a principal diagnosis of congestive heart failure (CHF) and with at least two determinations of patient weight and serum sodium, potassium, blood urea nitrogen (BUN), and creatinine levels (Figure 13).[20,**]

---

* The Joint Commission Obstetrical Care Indicator Development Task Force developed the following indicator, which is currently in the beta phase of field testing: "patients with excessive maternal blood loss defined by intra- and/or postpartum red blood cell transfusion or a low postdelivery hematocrit or hemoglobin (hematocrit less than 22%, hemoglobin less than 7 grams) or a significant pre- to postdelivery decrease in hematocrit (greater than or equal to 11%) or hemoglobin (greater than or equal to 3.5 grams), excluding patients with abruptio placenta or placenta previa."

† The Joint Commission Obstetrical Care Indicator Development Task Force developed the following indicator, which is currently in the beta phase of field testing: "patients with attempted vaginal birth after cesarean section (VBAC), subcategorized by success or failure."

‡ The Joint Commission Oncology Care Indicator Development Task Force developed the following indicator, which is currently in the beta phase of field testing: "patients with resections of primary colorectal cancer whose preoperative evaluation by a managing physician includes examination of the entire colon, liver function tests, chest x-ray, and carcinoembryonic antigen (CEA) levels."

§ The Joint Commission Trauma Care Indicator Development Task Force developed the following indicator, which is currently in the beta phase of field testing: "trauma patients with prehospital emergency medical services (EMS) scene times greater than 20 minutes."

** The Joint Commission Cardiovascular Care Indicator Development Task Force developed the following indicator, which is currently in the beta phase of field testing: "patients with a principal discharge diagnosis of congestive heart failure (CHF) and with at least two determinations of patient weight and of serum sodium, potassium, blood urea nitrogen (BUN), and creatinine levels."

136   Chapter 7

Figure 8

Joint Commission Beta Report Control Chart for Obstetrical Care Indicator:
"Patients with Primary Cesarean Section for Failure to Progress"*

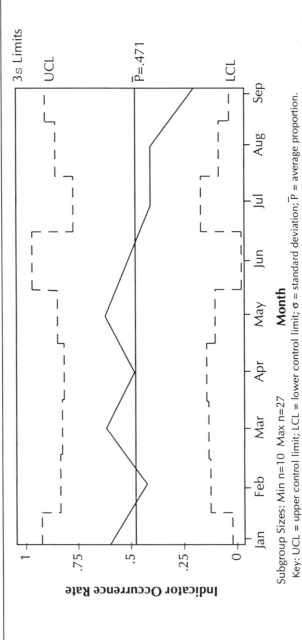

Subgroup Sizes: Min n=10 Max n=27

Key: UCL = upper control limit; LCL = lower control limit; σ = standard deviation; P̄ = average proportion.

Reporting period January 1, 1991, through September 30, 1991. Adapted from Joint Commission on Accreditation of Healthcare Organizations: *Beta I Feedback Reports: Obstetrical Care Indicators: 1991, Quarters I, II, III.* Oakbrook Terrace, IL, 1992, p 70.

Figure 9

Joint Commission Beta Report Control Chart for Obstetrical Care Indicator:

"Patients with Excessive Maternal Blood Loss"*

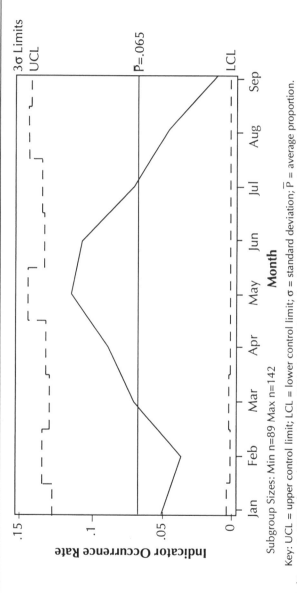

Subgroup Sizes: Min n=89 Max n=142

Key: UCL = upper control limit; LCL = lower control limit; σ = standard deviation; P̄ = average proportion.

*Reporting period January 1, 1991, through September 30, 1991. Adapted from Joint Commission on Accreditation of Healthcare Organizations: *Beta I Feedback Reports: Obstetrical Care Indicators: 1991, Quarters I, II, III.* Oakbrook Terrace, IL, 1992, p 76.

Figure 10

Joint Commission Beta Report Control Chart for Obstetrical Care Indicator:
"Patients with Successful Vaginal Birth After Cesarean Section"*

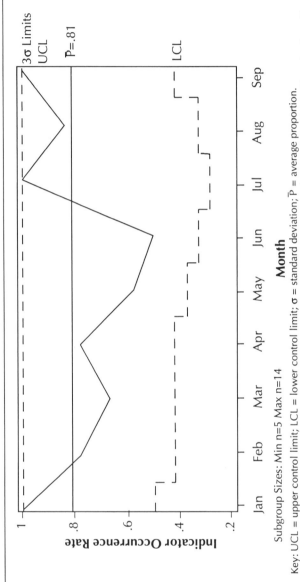

Subgroup Sizes: Min n=5 Max n=14

Key: UCL = upper control limit; LCL = lower control limit; σ = standard deviation; P̄ = average proportion.
*Reporting period January 1, 1991, through September 30, 1991. Adapted from Joint Commission on Accreditation of Healthcare Organizations: *Beta I Feedback Reports: Obstetrical Care Indicators: 1991, Quarters I, II, III.* Oakbrook Terrace, IL, 1992, p 74.

Figure 11

Joint Commission Beta Phase Control Chart for Oncology Indicator:

"Patients with Resections of Primary Colorectal Cancer Whose Preoperative Evaluation by a Managing Physician Includes Examination of the Entire Colon, Liver Function Tests, Chest X-ray, and Carcinoembryonic Antigen (CEA) Levels"*

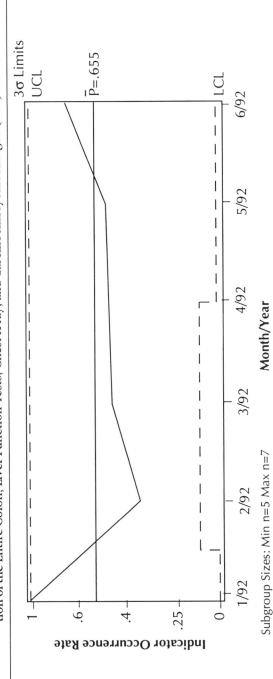

Subgroup Sizes: Min n=5 Max n=7

Key: UCL = upper control limit; LCL = lower control limit; σ = standard deviation; P̄ = average proportion.

*Reporting period January 1, 1992, through June 30, 1992. Adapted from Joint Commission on Accreditation of Healthcare Organizations: *Beta II Feedback Report: Oncology Indicators: 1992, Quarters I & II.* Oakbrook Terrace, IL, 1992, p 47.

Figure 12

Joint Commission Beta Report for Trauma Indicator:
"Trauma Patients with Prehospital Emergency Medical Services (EMS) Scene Times Greater than 20 Minutes"**

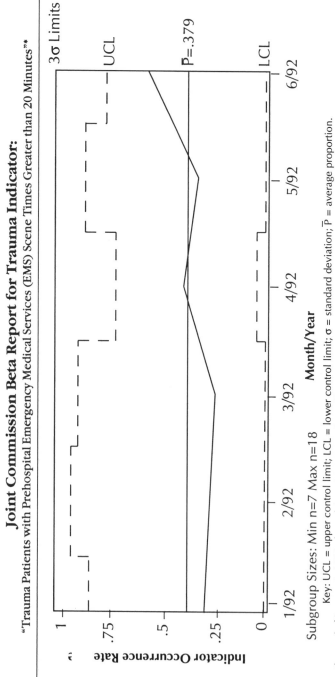

Subgroup Sizes: Min n=7 Max n=18

Key: UCL = upper control limit; LCL = lower control limit; σ = standard deviation; P̄ = average proportion.

*Reporting period January 1, 1992, through June 30, 1992. Adapted from Joint Commission on Accreditation of Healthcare Organizations: *Beta II Feedback Report: Trauma Indicators: 1992, Quarters I & II.* Oakbrook Terrace, IL, 1992, p 43.

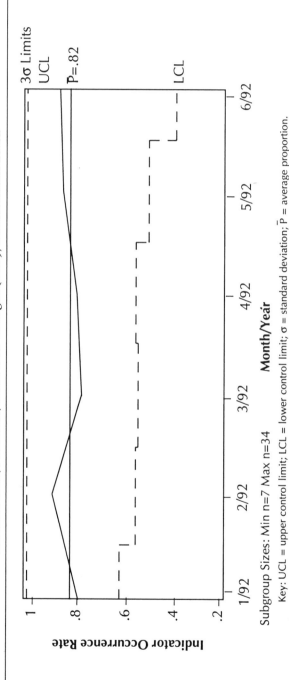

Figure 13

Joint Commission Beta Report for Cardiovascular Indicator:

"Patients with a Principal Diagnosis of Congestive Heart Failure (CHF) and with at Least Two Determinations of Patient Weight and Serum Sodium, Potassium, Blood Urea Nitrogen (BUN), and Creatinine Levels"*

Subgroup Sizes: Min n=7 Max n=34

Key: UCL = upper control limit; LCL = lower control limit; σ = standard deviation; P̄ = average proportion.

*Reporting period January 1, 1992, through June 30, 1992. Adapted from Joint Commission on Accreditation of Healthcare Organizations: *Beta II Feedback Report: Cardiovascular Indicators: 1992, Quarters I & II.* Oakbrook Terrace, IL, 1992, p 47.

One important reason why aggregate data indicators are so useful is that their relatively large numerators lend themselves easily to comparative analysis, while those indicators with small numerators (as in sentinel event indicators) are not as well suited to the use of helpful statistical tools and techniques. These techniques include, for instance, developing control charts such as those depicted in Figures 8 through 13. The results of statistical analyses can include intraorganizational and interorganizational comparative data that can be used for benchmarking and other performance improvement activities.

Sentinel event performance measures, in contrast to aggregate data indicators, identify unexpected events that organizations must always investigate because of the potential seriousness of the event for the patient, his or her family, practitioners, the organization, and the community. A sentinel event related to the urinary catheter use indicator previously described might be a patient death due to urosepsis in a postsurgical patient with a catheter.

The creation of useful health care performance databases has become urgent in recent years as the users of health care services increasingly demand accurate and complete data and information on which to base health care decisions. Sentinel event performance measures typically identify rare events such as maternal death and often are unable to generate prospectively useful data or information in the time frame currently mandated.

The second important characteristic of an aggregate data indicator is that it can express data about either a process or an outcome.[21] Indicators that measure the frequency of occurrence of use of indwelling urinary catheters for greater than 48 hours in perioperative patients undergoing selected surgical operations, or patients with principal discharge diagnosis of congestive heart failure with a documented etiology and chest x-ray substantiation of congestive heart failure, are *rate-based, process indicators.*[*,†]

---

* The Joint Commission Infection Control Indicator Development Task Force developed the following indicator, which is currently in the beta phase of field testing: "selected surgical procedures on inpatients who are catheterized during the perioperative period."

† The Joint Commission Cardiovascular Care Indicator Development Task Force developed the following indicator, which is currently in the beta phase of field testing: "patients with principal discharge diagnosis of congestive heart failure (CHF) with documented etiology and chest x-ray substantiation of CHF."

Indicators that measure the frequency of occurrence of intrahospital mortality of patients with principal discharge diagnosis of acute myocardial infarction, subcategorized by history of previous infarction, age, and intrahospital location of death, or patients undergoing pulmonary resection for primary lung cancer with postoperative complication of empyema, bronchopleural fistula, reoperation for postoperative bleeding, mechanical ventilation greater than five days postoperatively, or intrahospital death, are *rate-based, outcome indicators.*[*,†]

The ability of aggregate data indicators to measure both processes *and* outcomes is helpful to many organizations that have until recently focused exclusively on measurement of outcomes such as patient mortality. There are circumstances described in Chapter One for which process measurement is not only desirable but may be the only practical means for determining organizational performance. Sentinel event performance measures tend to focus solely on outcomes.

A third important characteristic of an aggregate data indicator is its ability to provide organizations with an early warning of performance areas requiring attention. This characteristic does not often apply to sentinel event performance measures.

Compare, for instance, the rate-based indicator:

Patients with *life-threatening cardiac dysrhythmias* during or within one postprocedure day of procedures involving anesthesia administration, excluding patients with required intraoperative cardiac arrest, subcategorized by American Society of Anesthesiologists Physical Status (ASA-PS) class, patient

---

* The Joint Commission Cardiovascular Care Indicator Development Task Force developed the following indicator, which is currently in the beta phase of field testing: "intrahospital mortality of patients with principal discharge diagnosis of acute myocardial infarction, subcategorized by history of previous infarction, age, and intrahospital location of death."

† The Joint Commission Oncology Care Indicator Development Task Force developed the following indicator, which is currently in the beta phase of field testing: "patients undergoing pulmonary resection for primary lung cancer with postoperative complication of empyema, bronchopleural fistula, reoperation for postoperative bleeding, mechanical ventilation greater than five days postoperatively, or intrahospital death."

age, and cardiac versus noncardiac procedures,"

and the sentinel event performance measure:

> *Patients with cardiac arrest* during or within one postprocedure
> day of procedures involving anesthesia administration, exclud-
> ing patients with required intraoperative cardiac arrest,
> subcategorized by ASA-PS class, patient age, and cardiac versus
> noncardiac procedures.*

Life-threatening cardiac dysrhythmias, such as ventricular
tachycardia and ventricular fibrillation, often precede, but do not
necessarily result in, cardiac asystole and death, especially when
dysrhythmias are effectively managed. Use of a rate-based indicator
dealing with cardiac dysrhythmias can provide data that inform an
organization about the potential need for performance improvement
in this area. An unacceptably high rate of cardiac dysrhythmias—
even in the absence of a single cardiac arrest occurrence—would tell
the organization that it must investigate further to determine reasons
why the rate is higher than expected. The rate gives the organization
time to address underlying issues *before* cardiac arrests follow
dysrhythmias. Such indicators can be used as tools to aid in the
prevention of less frequently occurring events such as death or
debilitating complications of care.

Use of a sentinel event performance measure dealing with the
occurrence of cardiac arrests, by contrast, informs the organization
after the fact that an undesirable and potentially avoidable patient
health outcome has occurred. Although the organization is triggered
by the occurrence of this event to investigate and correct underlying
causes, potentially avoidable and undesirable outcomes such as death
have already occurred.

*A fourth characteristic of an aggregate data indicator is that it can
express data about occurrences that are either desirable or undesirable.*[21]
Patients who develop nosocomial pneumonia, live neonates with a
discharge diagnosis of significant birth trauma, and patients with
excessive maternal blood loss are *undesirable* events measurable by
aggregate data indicators. Patients with attempted vaginal birth after

---

* The Joint Commission Anesthesia Care Indicator Development Task Force
developed this indicator, which is currently in the beta phase of field testing.

previous cesarean section and patients with successful vaginal birth after previous cesarean section are usually *desirable* events measurable by aggregate data indicators.

The ability of aggregate data indicators to measure desirable occurrences is a welcome respite from earlier quality assurance approaches that focused almost exclusively on problem detection and correction. Sentinel event performance measures of that era typically identified undesirable occurrences that often represented the most extreme examples of flawed care. Indicators that measure the good things accomplished by organizations are especially well-suited to the continuous improvement paradigm currently being embraced by many health care organizations.[22–24]

A fifth characteristic of an aggregate data indicator is its ability to express data that guide organizations in improving their norms of performance instead of focusing exclusively on censoring or eliminating individual outliers.[22] Quantitative performance data, when properly disseminated, can have an "immense and irresistible power in shifting the entire curve of [organizational performance] upward. . . ."[22] The power of credible data to change and improve practice patterns and organizational systems of care is at the heart of many performance improvement initiatives today, including the Joint Commission's beta phase of indicator testing, which is designed to test indicators in preparation for implementation of an indicator monitoring system. Aggregate data indicators help identify patterns (for example, helping to differentiate common cause from special cause variation), which sentinel event performance measures generally cannot do.

Many organizations are finding that performance improvement objectives can be achieved better when attention is paid to lifting the performance levels of the majority of staff members who invariably enjoy learning and improving their own performance and that of their units. When an organization dwells exclusively on finding, blaming, and rooting out deficient individuals, departments, or disciplines, its attention is also diverted away from the essential need to measure, assess, and improve everyday processes, systems, and functions.

Development of Indicators—Lessons Learned

Approaches to the development and validation of indicators—especially rate-based indicators—are described in detail in *Primer on*

Indicator Development and Application.[25] An overview of the Joint Commission's current Indicator Development Form, which contains each indicator's complete information set, is reproduced in Appendix D. An example of a completed form is depicted in Appendix E. Here we summarize important lessons learned by organizations and groups involved in developing indicators (see Table 10).

The first lesson is that the literature on organizational performance, including data comparing performance among institutions, multihospital performance, and performance of an everyday nature, is extremely sparse. Groups and individuals that pursue expensive, time-consuming literature searches and reviews often come up relatively empty-handed simply because performance of an everyday nature has not been well-studied in the past. Where studies on the same subject do actually exist, widely variable results are common, leading to more dilemmas as to deciding which researchers and/or data to accept. Considerable statistical expertise is often required to determine the validity of methodologies used to obtain the study results.

Many indicator development groups that have experienced an unsatisfying literature search choose to convene a panel of experts to develop indicators through the process of expert consensus. Expert consensus as to what constitutes a valid indicator may lack scientific rigor, but its work products are likely to enjoy credibility, at least in the beginning stages of performance measurement efforts. Approaches to selecting methodology and content experts that can make up an expert panel are described in detail elsewhere.[25]

A second lesson is that a multidisciplinary, multidepartmental team approach to indicator development increases the probability that meaningful indicators will evolve to meet the need for which they are being created—that is, improving organizational performance and the quality of services provided to patients and other users of services. This means that representatives from *all* relevant areas of the organization should be included in the indicator development process. Medical staff especially should be actively included in the process of developing indicators designed to improve patient health services and outcomes. Insufficient physician involvement in the indicator development process, for whatever reasons, is a serious and growing concern among individuals experienced in the performance measurement, assessment, and improvement function.[26-27] The multidisciplinary,

Table 10

Lessons Learned During Development of Indicators

- The literature on organizational performance is sparse.
- A multidisciplinary, multidepartmental team approach to indicator development increases the probability that meaningful indicators will evolve to meet the need for which they are being created—that is, improving organizational performance and the quality of services provided to patients and other users of services.
- Professional instincts and experience often result in development of a predominance of sentinel event performance measures even though this type of measures has certain limitations. Education about the need to develop aggregate data indicators is usually sufficient to offset a tendency to develop a predominance of sentinel event indicators.
- Many health professionals lack rudimentary knowledge about information management issues such as data element accuracy and completeness.
- Organizations involved in any performance database should be knowledgeable about exactly how these databases work to produce performance measurement data.
- Indicator parsimony is a necessary precondition for indicator data and information parsimony.

multidepartmental team approach to indicator development may be novel and even threatening to many, but it unquestionably supports the best interests of patients.

A third lesson is that professional instincts and experience often result in development of a predominance of sentinel event performance measures even though this type of measure is not as useful as aggregate data measures within a performance measurement, assessment, and improvement framework. Sentinel event performance measures often identify the most egregious examples of ineffective, inappropriate, or unsafe care and have commonly provided the substrate for traditional morbidity and mortality conferences.

Most groups developing indicators will benefit from education about aggregate data indicators. Aggregate data indicators can be used to identify patterns in care, and professionals steadily come to understand that appropriate interventions designed to promote desired patterns can be effective in forestalling the rare occurrences upon which their (and sentinel event indicators') attention was originally focused. Effective and informed leadership is indispensible in steering a group away from the development of sentinel event performance measures, toward the development of aggregate data indicators.

A fourth lesson learned is that many health professionals lack rudimentary knowledge about information management issues such as data element accuracy and completeness. A group of professionals may recommend the collection of many important and useful data elements, some of which can be easily collected and others which cannot be easily collected. Data elements in the latter category include those that may be haphazardly documented and stored somewhere in the organization or those that are prohibitively expensive to collect.

Members of an indicator development group often develop a keen appetite to learn more about the spectrum of data issues, especially as they relate to the measurement, assessment, and improvement of organizational performance. The inclusion in indicator development groups of an information management specialist with good interpersonal communication and teaching skills can help the process of educating health professionals about data issues they may likely encounter.

A fifth lesson learned is that organizations involved in any performance database should be knowledgeable about exactly how these databases work to produce performance measurement data. Information on how performance data are derived (the process by which inputs such as data elements are transformed into outputs such as performance information) should be reasonably accessible and understandable to interested persons or groups.[28]

There is a growing concern that medical information systems that produce performance information may rely on a "black box," defined as "any unknown system, especially one considered solely in terms of input and output, without an understanding of its workings."[29-30] How inputs are transformed into outputs in these black boxes may be kept secret for proprietary reasons or may be incomprehensible.[29-30] This places users of the data in a precarious situation because they cannot confirm the validity of performance data and information that have been issued.

A sixth lesson learned is that indicator parsimony is a necessary precondition for indicator data and information parsimony. A multidisciplinary, multidepartmental group of individuals convened to develop indicators in a performance area can easily become so enthusiastic in their efforts that they develop more indicators than the organization can possibly handle, at least at the outset. Two sayings iterated several years ago bear repeating here: Ultimately, organizations and the staff members who serve in them must be masters of data, not slaves to data. And health care organizations should collect only data that are needed and use all data that are collected.[31]

The Third Step: Using Measurement Instruments

The third step of a performance measurement system consists of *using* the measurement instrument to quantify the extent to which a process or an outcome possesses the performance attribute under study. The actual use of aggregate data indicators now encompasses a large and growing area of knowledge and expertise.

An important component of the Joint Commission's Agenda for Change initiative, for instance, is the development of an indicator-based performance monitoring system for accredited health care organizations. This system, sometimes called the "indicator monitoring system," is designed to:

- Continuously collect objective data, which are derived from the application of aggregate data indicators, with respect to the performance of important processes, systems, or functions, and the achievement of important outcomes by each accredited health care organization;
- Aggregate, risk adjust as necessary, and analyze the performance data on a national level;
- Provide comparative performance data to accredited health care organizations for use in their internal performance improvement efforts;
- Identify patterns in the performance of individual accredited health care organizations that may call for more focused attention at the organizational level; and

- Provide a national performance database that can serve as a resource for health services research.[32]

How are aggregate data indicators used by accredited organizations and the Joint Commission to generate reliable and valid performance data and information? This process involves data element collection followed by reaggregation of data elements through use of specific indicator logic to produce indicator occurrence rates.

Collection of Indicator Data Elements

Indicators have been described as groups of data elements that define a given indicator's precision or generality and can, to a certain extent, address risk adjustment needs of organizations.[33] Data elements are generally dates, times, coded character values, and numbers. They are the raw building blocks of indicator occurrence rate calculation. Data elements for each indicator will be collected and transmitted on a voluntary basis in 1994 by accredited health care organizations to the Joint Commission for analysis.

Consider, for instance, the rate-based indicator, "inpatients receiving parenteral aminoglycosides who have a measured aminoglycoside serum level," developed by the Joint Commission Medication Use Indicator Development Task Force and currently undergoing field study at hundreds of hospitals.[34] The required data elements for data collection are

1. birthdate of patient   mm/dd/yy
2. patient receiving aminoglycoside   yes/no
3. aminoglycoside serum drug level drawn   yes/no
4. aminoglycoside given prophylactically   yes/no

The fourth data element—"aminoglycoside given prophylactically"—is required because patients receiving prophylactic aminoglycosides need not have a measured serum level; inclusion of these patients may contribute to a low rate.[34] An indicator's required data elements should be listed in the Indicator Development Form under the section titled "Required Data Elements for Data Collection" (see Appendix E).

A second example involves the rate-based indicator, "patients less than 25 years old with a principal discharge diagnosis of bronchoconstrictive pulmonary disease, who are readmitted to the hospital or visit the emergency department within 15 days of discharge due to an exacerbation of their principal diagnosis," also developed by the Joint Commission Medication Use Indicator Development Task Force and currently undergoing field testing.[35] The data elements required for data collection are

1. birthdate   mm/dd/yy
2. type of return visit   emergency department admission

   no visit
3. date of return visit   mm/dd/yy
4. is reason for return visit related to respiratory (breathing) problem   yes/no
5. discharge date of last hospitalization   mm/dd/yy
6. principal ICD-9-CM discharge diagnostic code of last hospitalization _____._

A master list of data elements for an indicator set—that is, a group of related indicators such as medication use indicators—is often assembled for reference. The master lists currently being used during beta testing of the Joint Commission's medication use and infection control indicator sets are reproduced in Appendix F. These master lists are in testing, and the final master lists for the Joint Commission's indicator monitoring system may differ.

The data elements in the Joint Commission's beta phase of indicator testing are collected manually (by longhand) or through organizational computer systems. Manual collection is accomplished through use of a manual data collection form. Two examples of this form are depicted in Figures 14 and 15 for the indicators, "inpatients receiving parenteral aminoglycosides who have a measured aminoglycoside serum level" and "patients less than 25 years old with a principal diagnosis of bronchoconstrictive pulmonary disease, who are readmitted to the hospital or visit the emergency department within 15 days of discharge due to an exacerbation of their principal diagnosis," respectively.

Computerized collection of data elements is accomplished through use of computer software, called the Indicator Development Entry System (IDES), developed specifically for use by accredited health care organizations and the Joint Commission in the beta testing phase for some indicators. The IDES is an information management system designed to be used by hospitals for independent self-analysis

---

Figure 14

Manual Data Collection Form for Medication Use Indicator:

"Inpatients Receiving Parenteral Aminoglycosides Who Have a Measured Aminoglycoside Serum Level"*

Medication Use—Form A Section 1 Data Elements

Complete the following information for the selected patient.

Note: It is necessary that you provide the information below.

Medical Record Number
☐☐☐☐☐☐☐☐☐☐☐☐☐☐☐☐☐☐

Sample Date: Admission Date: Discharge Date:
M M D D Y Y   M M D D Y Y   M M D D Y Y
☐☐/☐☐/☐☐   ☐☐/☐☐/☐☐   ☐☐/☐☐/☐☐

---

1. Patient's First Name: ☐☐☐☐☐☐☐☐☐☐☐☐☐☐☐

2. Patient's Last Name: ☐☐☐☐☐☐☐☐☐☐☐☐☐☐☐

Indicate whether the patient was receiving one or more of the following three aminoglycosides: Tobramycin, Gentamicin, and/or Amikacin.

Excluding: Streptomycin, Neomycin, and Paramycin

3. Is The Patient Receiving an Aminoglycoside?

❑ 1= Yes ——▶ After completing this section, also complete Section 2.
❑ 2= No

Indicate whether the patient is receiving one or more of the following medications.

4. Is Patient Receiving Digoxin? (excluding digitoxin derivatives)

❑ 1= Yes ——▶ After completing this section, also complete Section 3.
❑ 2= No

5. Is Patient Receiving Theophylline? (excluding all theophylline derivatives, see definition of terms for a comprehensive list)

❑ 1= Yes ——▶ After completing this section, also complete Section 3.
❑ 2= No

GO TO NEXT PAGE

---

*This indicator was developed by the Joint Commission Medication Use Indicator Development Task Force.

Figure 14 (continued)

Manual Data Collection Form for Medication Use Indicator:

"Inpatients Receiving Parenteral Aminoglycosides Who Have a Measured Aminoglycoside Serum Level"*

Medication Use—Form A Section 2 Data Elements

Complete the following information for patients who received an aminoglycoside.

Note: | It is necessary that you provide the information below.

Medical Record Number
☐☐☐☐☐☐☐☐☐☐☐☐☐☐☐☐☐

Patient's First Name: ☐☐☐☐☐☐☐☐☐☐☐☐☐☐☐

Patient's Last Name: ☐☐☐☐☐☐☐☐☐☐☐☐☐☐

Admission Date: Discharge Date:
M M D D Y Y   M M D D Y Y
☐☐/☐☐/☐☐   ☐☐/☐☐/☐☐

---

11. Was Aminoglycoside Given Prophylactically?

   ❑ 1= Yes
   ❑ 2= No

12. Was a Serum Aminoglycoside Level Drawn?
   ❑ 1= Yes
   ❑ 2= No

END OF SECTION 2

---

*This indicator was developed by the Joint Commission Medication Use Indicator Development Task Force.

Figure 15

Manual Data Collection Form for Medication Use Indicator:

"Patients Less than 25 Years Old with a Principal Diagnosis of Bronchoconstrictive Pulmonary Disease, Who Are Readmitted to the Hospital or Visit the Emergency Department Within 15 Days of Discharge Due to an Exacerbation of Their Principal Diagnosis"*

Medication Use—Form C Data Elements

Note: Complete this section if patient is less than 25 years old and has a principal ICD–9–CM discharge diagnosis code equal to:

491.0, 491.1, 491.2-, 492.8, 493.00, 493.01, 493.10, 493.11, 493.20, 493.21, 493.90, 493.91, 466.0 + 491.2-, 491.2- +518.82, 518.81+ 491.2-, 518.81+ 493.2-, 518.81+ 496., 518.82 + 492.8

AND

if patient is listed on concurrent tracking worksheet from Emergency Department or Admitting Department

Note: It is necessary that you provide the information below.

Medical Record Number
□□□□□□□□□□□□□□□□□□

Patient's First Name: □□□□□□□□□□□□□□□□

Patient's Last Name: □□□□□□□□□□□□□□□□

Birthdate: Admission Date: Discharge Date:
M M D D Y E A R   M M D D Y Y   M M D D Y Y
□□/□□/□□□□   □□/□□/□□   □□/□□/□□

Sampling Period: _____
(Enter in free form text.)

---

102. Type of Return Visit:

  ❏ 1= Emergency Department
      (If patient is admitted through Emergency Department, **select 2**)
  ❏ 2= Admission
  ❏ 3= No Visit

103. Date of Return Visit:
M M D D Y Y
□□/□□/□□

104. Is This Patient's Reason for Return Visit Related to Respiratory (breathing) Problems?

  ❏ 1= Yes
  ❏ 2= No

END OF DATA COLLECTION FORM C

---

*This indicator was developed by the Joint Commission Medication Use Indicator Development Task Force.

as well as to provide data elements for transfer to the Joint Commission for national comparative analysis during the beta phase of indicator testing. The system presents a framework in which an organization can combine data and customize reports to present information in the way that meets its needs.

The IDES can transmit data elements required for submission to the Joint Commission via modem or diskette. In some cases IDES maintains more information than is needed by the Joint Commission. These data, such as patient medical record numbers and identities of attending physicians, are intended for hospital use only. They *are not* included in the transmission to the Joint Commission.

In addition to the raw indicator data elements that are collected and transmitted by organizations, there are calculated data elements. These data elements are calculated by the IDES at the time of data entry or download. They include frequently referenced combinations of data elements that are calculated for convenience, such as the number of hours in the emergency department, the number of days from a percutaneous transluminal coronary artery procedure to discharge, or the first available and last available Glasgow Coma Scores. They also include "housekeeping" data elements such as the date of last record update or missing data element status.

Once the indicator data elements have been transmitted by accredited organizations to the Joint Commission, analysis and reaggregation of the data elements are performed to determine specific indicator occurrence rates. The analytic process flows according to precise aggregation rules sometimes referred to as "Indicator Data Entry System Logic" or IDES logic.

Indicator Data Entry System Logic

There is a logic or flow of general steps that is required to establish indicator occurrence rates from data elements. Individual health care organizations can perform this exercise for each indicator; it is also performed by the IDES.

This logic is flowcharted using standard flowchart symbols to depict the processes and decisions required to define the indicator event. An example of this flowcharting is depicted in Figure 16 for the indicator, "inpatients receiving parenteral aminoglycosides who have a measured aminoglycoside serum level" and in Figure 17 for the indicator, "patients less than 25 years old with a principal diagnosis

---

Figure 16

Indicator Logic for Medication Use Indicator:
"Inpatients Receiving Parenteral Aminoglycosides Who Have a
Measured Aminoglycoside Serum Level"*

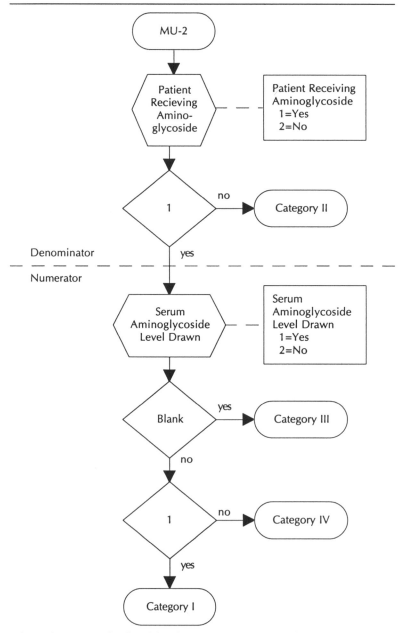

*This indicator was developed by the Joint Commission Medication Use Indicator Development Task Force.

of bronchoconstrictive pulmonary disease, who are readmitted to the hospital or visit the emergency department within 15 days of discharge due to an exacerbation of their principal diagnosis.*, †

The IDES software logic assigns a category—category 1 through category 5—to each case evaluated by the indicator.[36]

Category 1 means there are insufficient data to determine whether the record is a member of the population referenced by the indicator (the denominator population). Eligibility of the case for inclusion in the indicator occurrence rate is undetermined because key data elements that determine if the case meets criteria for consideration are missing from the database.

Category 2 means the record is not a member of the denominator population referenced by the indicator. The record is therefore ineligible because sufficient data elements are in the database to determine that the case does not meet the criteria for the specified indicator.

Category 3 means the record is a member of the reference (denominator) population but more data are needed to fully classify the record. The record has potential numerator eligibility because sufficient data elements are present to determine that the case is in the denominator, but there are insufficient data to determine if the case is an indicator event.

Category 4 means the record is a member of the reference (denominator) population for the indicator, but it lacks the outcome characteristics that were measured, and it therefore is not an indicator event; the case is a denominator case only. The record has an eligible denominator, meaning sufficient data are present to determine that the case belongs in the denominator.

Category 5 means the record is a member of the indicator reference population and has the characteristics that were measured by the indicator (numerator as well as denominator case). This record is an indicator-identified case, meaning that sufficient data are present to determine that the case meets the criteria for an indicator event.

---

* The Joint Commission Medication Use Indicator Development Task Force developed this indicator, which is currently in the beta phase of field testing.

† The Joint Commission Medication Use Indicator Development Task Force developed this indicator, which is currently in the beta phase of field testing.

Figure 17

Indicator Logic for Medication Use Indicator:
"Patients Less than 25 Years Old with a Principal Diagnosis of Bronchoconstrictive Pulmonary Disease, Who Are Readmitted to the Hospital or Visit the Emergency Department Within 15 Days of Discharge Due to an Exacerbation of Their Principal Diagnosis."*

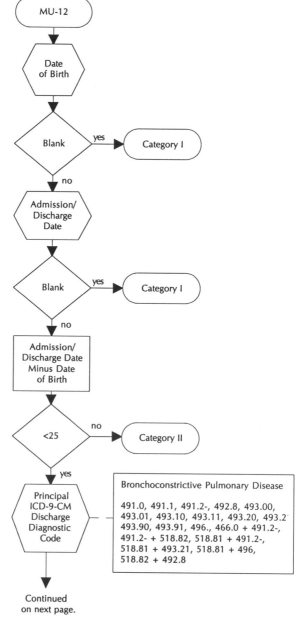

Continued
on next page.

*This indicator was developed by the Joint Commission Medication Use Indicator Development Task Force.

Figure 17 (continued)

Indicator Logic for Medication Use Indicator:

"Patients Less than 25 Years Old with a Principal Diagnosis of Bronchoconstrictive Pulmonary Disease, Who Are Readmitted to the Hospital or Visit the Emergency Department Within 15 Days of Discharge Due to an Exacerbation of Their Principal Diagnosis."*

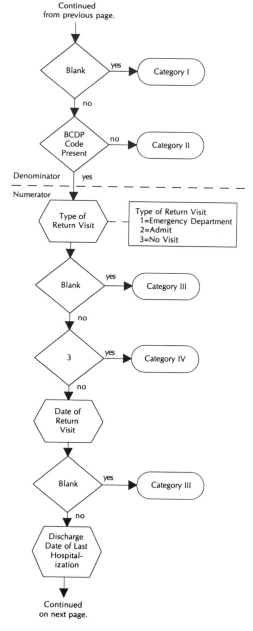

*This indicator was developed by the Joint Commission Medication Use Indicator Development Task Force.

_____

Figure 17 (continued)

Indicator Logic for Medication Use Indicator:

"Patients Less than 25 Years Old with a Principal Diagnosis of Bronchoconstrictive Pulmonary Disease, Who Are Readmitted to the Hospital or Visit the Emergency Department Within 15 Days of Discharge Due to an Exacerbation of Their Principal Diagnosis."*

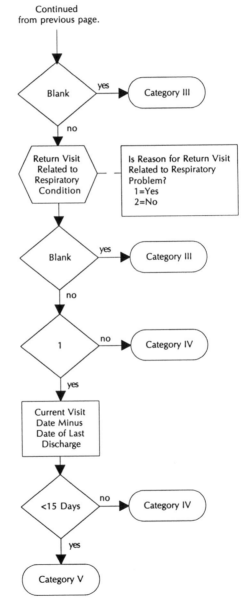

*This indicator was developed by the Joint Commission Medication Use Indicator Development Task Force.

When analyzing indicator rates, users should restrict the reports to include only cases that are in categories 4 or 5. Typically indicator occurrence rates are calculated as follows:

$$\frac{\text{All category 5 cases}}{\text{All category 4 cases} + \text{All category 5 cases}}$$

Indicator Reliability and Validity Testing

The degree to which performance data are accurate and complete is important because of the broad range of processes and activities that are subsequently conducted based on these data. Indicators must be rigorously tested for their degrees of reliability and validity and constantly improved whenever necessary to ensure that performance data are credible and trustworthy for users.

Reliability and validity testing of indicators being developed under the aegis of the Joint Commission occurs during the alpha and beta testing phases of indicator development. Reliability testing involves the quantification of the accuracy and completeness with which indicator occurrences are identified from among all cases at risk of being indicator occurrences.[37] Reliability testing answers the question: "Does the indicator correctly identify the event that has been targeted for monitoring?"[38] This evaluation addresses the adequacy of indicator design as well as the potential problems of incorrect or missing data elements.

Validity testing involves quantification of the extent to which indicators identify events that merit further review by various individuals or groups providing or affecting the process or outcome of care defined by the indicator.[37] Validity testing answers the questions: "Do the occurrences identified by the indicator merit further review? Does the indicator raise substantive questions about performance?"[38]

The Joint Commission has invested heavily in the reliability and validity testing of the indicators developed by its expert task forces. Joint Commission staff members, for instance, are currently involved with a subset of beta test site hospitals asked to participate in the reliability and validity component of the indicator development process. The onsite activities of staff members include the following:

- Reabstraction of selected data elements that were transmitted to the Joint Commission;
- Identification of factors that appear to be related to inaccurately identified indicator events;
- Assessment of the ability of the indicator(s) to identify cases that represent potential opportunities to improve care or services; and
- Collection of opinions and recommendations regarding the ability of the indicators to portray organizational performance and to provide useful information to the Joint Commission as a part of the monitoring process.[38]

Additional information about the Joint Commission's approach to indicator reliability and validity testing is available elsewhere.[37–38]

Beyond Performance Measurement

Performance measurement is the first segment in the trilogy of performance measurement, performance assessment, and performance improvement. Performance assessment is the process by which data generated by performance measurement activities are analyzed and interpreted. Performance assessment involves, among other processes, the application of statistical tools and techniques to the database to provide health care organizations with graphs such as the control charts depicted in Figures 8 through 13. These control charts can be used to make decisions regarding performance improvement opportunities.

A rigorous approach to performance measurement is imperative because the success enjoyed by performance assessment and improvement based on data ultimately depends on the quality of data resulting from performance measurement efforts.

Summary Observations

Performance measurement involves a logical sequence of activities. There are several important observations about this sequence that bear emphasis.

1. A performance measurement system is composed of three steps: establishment of units of measure, development and validation of instruments capable of quantifying the units of measure, and use of the instruments to produce measurement data for subsequent analysis.

2. Establishment of units of measure may be challenging for many reasons, including the need to shift from using subjective human perception alone to judge level of performance to using units of measure to quantify level of performance; variation in opinions as to what constitutes a valid unit of measure; and public demand for performance data within a relatively short time frame. A functions-oriented approach to establishing units of measure can facilitate this process.

3. Aggregate data indicators are performance measurement instruments with many important characteristics. Aggregate data indicators are based on collection and aggregation of data about many events or phenomena. The events or phenomena may be desirable or undesirable, and the data may be reported as a continuous variable or as a discrete variable.

4. A rate-based indicator (also called a discrete variable indicator) is an aggregate data indicator in which the value of each measurement is expressed as a proportion or a ratio. A continuous variable indicator is also an aggregate data indicator in which the value of each measurement can fall anywhere along a continuous scale (for example, the number of inches, or length, of sticks).

5. A sentinel event indicator identifies an individual event or phenomenon that always triggers further analysis and investigation each time the event or phenomenon occurs. The event or phenomenon measured by a sentinel event indicator usually occurs infrequently and is undesirable in nature. Sentinel event indicators are generally viewed as being of limited value because they represent the extremes of performance measurement.

6. Use of aggregate data indicators involves collection of indicator data elements either manually or via automated systems and application of indicator data entry system logic to generate indicator occurrence rates and other descriptions of the data.

7. Indicator validity and reliability testing is essential because a large number of activities are subsequently conducted based on the data expressed by indicators.

8. Performance measurement is the first segment in the trilogy of performance measurement, performance assessment, and performance improvement. A rigorous approach to performance measurement is imperative because the success enjoyed by performance assessment and performance improvement activities ultimately de-

pends on the quality of the performance data generated during the performance measurement phase.

References

1. *Juran's Quality Control Handbook* 4th ed. 1988. Juran JM (ed). New York: McGraw-Hill Book Company, p 18.57.

2. Ibid, p 18.56.

3. Gitlow H, et al. 1989. *Tools and Methods for Improvement of Quality.* Homewood, IL: Irwin, p 379.

4. Joint Commission on Accreditation of Healthcare Organizations. 1990. *Primer for Indicator Development and Application.* Oakbrook Terrace, IL, pp 12–14, 42–43.

5. Gitlow H, et al. 1989. *Tools and Methods for Improvement of Quality.* Homewood, IL: Irwin, pp 80–81.

6. Ibid, pp 290–291.

7. Hart JA. 1985. The urethral catheter: A review of its implication in urinary tract infection. *International J Nursing Studies* 22:57–70.

8. Mulhall AB, Chapman RG, Crow RA. 1988. Bacteriuria during indwelling urethral catheterization. *J Hosp Infect* 11:253–262.

9. Nickel JC, Grant SK, Scosterton JW. 1985. Catheter-associated bacteriuria. An experimental study. *Urology* 26:369–375.

10. Shapiro M, et al. 1984. A multivariant analysis of risk factors for acquiring bacteriuria in patients with indwelling urinary catheters for longer than twenty-four hours. *Am J Infect Control* 5:525–532.

11. Stickler DJ, Chawla JC. 1988. An appraisal of antibiotic policies for urinary tract infections in patients with spinal cord injuries undergoing long-term intermittent catheterization. *Paraplegia* 26:215–225.

12. Woods DR, Bender BS. 1989. Long-term urinary tract catheterization. *Med Clin North Am* 73:1441–1454.

13. Joint Commission on Accreditation of Healthcare Organizations. 1991. *Medication Use and Infection Control Indicators Beta Phase Training Manual and Software User's Guide.* Oakbrook Terrace, IL, pp 6.17–6.25.

14. Joint Commission on Accreditation of Healthcare Organizations. 1992. *Beta I Feedback Reports: Obstetrical Care Indicators: 1991, Quarters I,II,III.* Oakbrook Terrace, IL, pp 19–20.

15. Joint Commission on Accreditation of Healthcare Organizations. 1992. *Beta I Feedback Reports: Obstetrical Care Indicators: 1991, Quarters I,II,III.* Oakbrook Terrace, IL, p 70.

16. Ibid, p 76.

17. Ibid, p 74.

18. Joint Commission on Accreditation of Healthcare Organizations. 1992. *Beta II Feedback Reports: Oncology Indicators: 1992, Quarters I & II.* Oakbrook Terrace, IL, pp 46–47.

19. Joint Commission on Accreditation of Healthcare Organizations. 1992. *Beta II Feedback Reports: Trauma Indicators: 1992, Quarters I & II.* Oakbrook Terrace, IL, p 43.

20. Joint Commission on Accreditation of Healthcare Organizations. 1992. *Beta II Feedback Report: Cardiovascular Indicators: 1992, Quarters I & II.* Oakbrook Terrace, IL, pp 46–47.

21. Joint Commission on Accreditation of Healthcare Organizations. 1990. *Primer on Indicator Development and Application.* Oakbrook Terrace, IL, pp 10–11.

22. Berwick DM. 1989. Continuous improvement as an ideal in health care. *N Engl J Med* 320:53–56.

23. Kritchevsky SB, Simmons BP. 1991. Continuous quality improvement. *JAMA* 266:1817–1823.

24. Joint Commission on Accreditation of Healthcare Organizations. 1991. *An Introduction to Quality Improvement in Health Care.* Oakbrook Terrace, IL.

25. Joint Commission on Accreditation of Healthcare Organizations. 1990. *Primer on Indicator Development and Application.* Oakbrook Terrace, IL, p 28.

26. Joint Commission on Accreditation of Healthcare Organizations. 1991. *Striving Toward Improvement: Six Hospitals in Search of Quality.* Oakbrook Terrace, IL, pp 223–229.

27. MacInnes RM. 1992. Physician leaders and the transition of quality improvement. In Lord JT (ed). *The Physician Leader's Guide.* Rockville, MD, pp 39–44.

28. Joint Commission on Accreditation of Healthcare Organizations. 1991. *Development and Application of Indicators for Continuous Improvement in Surgical and Anesthesia Care.* Oakbrook Terrace, IL, p 17.

29. Iezzoni LI. 1991. "Black box" medical information systems: A technology needing assessment. *JAMA* 265:3006–3007.

30. Blumberg MS. 1991. Biased estimates of expected acute myocardial infarction mortality using MedisGroups admission severity groups. *JAMA* 265:2965–2970.

31. Joint Commission on Accreditation of Healthcare Organizations. 1990. *Primer on Indicator Development and Application.* Oakbrook Terrace, IL, p 35.

32. Joint Commission on Accreditation of Healthcare Organizations. 1991. *Medication Use and Infection Control Indicators Beta Phase Training Manual and Software User's Guide.* Oakbrook Terrace, IL, p 3.9.

33. O'Leary DS, O'Leary MR. 1992. From quality assurance to quality improvement. *Emergency Clinics of North America* 10:477–492.

34. Joint Commission on Accreditation of Healthcare Organizations. 1991. *Medication Use and Infection Control Indicators Beta Phase Training Manual and Software User's Guide.* Oakbrook Terrace, IL, pp 4.6–4.9.

35. Ibid, pp 4.64–4.71.

36. Ibid, p 3.23.

37. Joint Commission on Accreditation of Healthcare Organizations. 1990. *Primer on Indicator Development and Application.* Oakbrook Terrace, IL, pp 39–45.

38. Joint Commission on Accreditation of Healthcare Organizations. 1991. *Medication Use and Infection Control Indicators Beta Phase Trianing Manual and Software User's Guide.* Oakbrook Terrace, IL, pp 3.11–3.12.

·CHAPTER·

8

Case Studies in Performance Measurement

Performance measurement, assessment, and improvement require commitment of organizations' leadership to organizing, fostering, and supporting the efforts of individuals at all levels throughout the organization over time. These individuals must commonly cross boundaries to work with others to make progress toward improvement goals. The following case studies give practical insight into the mechanics and potential pitfalls of measuring performance.

CASE 1: Recognizing and Following Through on the Need to Measure Performance

Two new medical staff members of Hospital A, during the 1980s, express concerns about the effectiveness and appropriateness with which cardiopulmonary resuscitation (CPR) is being performed by house staff members, medical staff, nurses, and other health professionals. Specifically, these hospital personnel do not demonstrate a strong familiarity with emergency cardiac care treatment, such as the approach developed and taught by the American Heart Association.[1] The organizationwide, multidisciplinary character of this process leads the physicians to express their concerns to members of the hospital's quality assurance committee. One member of this com-

167

mittee duly notes that a group of organizational standards exist that express the expectation that "cardiopulmonary resuscitation training be conducted as often as necessary, but not less than annually, for appropriate . . . staff members who cannot otherwise document their competence."[2]

Committee members state that they are interested in investigating this process of care for at least two reasons: an accreditation survey is nigh, and functions-oriented approaches to performance improvement in health care organizations are being taught and recommended, according to the chief of internal medicine and a quality assurance staff member who recently attended a national meeting dealing with continuous quality improvement. A CPR task force composed of representatives of administration, anesthesiology, internal medicine, nursing, obstetrics and gynecology, pediatrics, pharmaceutical services, respiratory therapy, and surgery, is appointed to "find out what we know" about the organization's performance effectiveness and appropriateness in carrying out CPR.

The task force spends three months obtaining information about the performance of CPR in the institution. The following results of the investigation are reported at the monthly meeting of the hospital's quality assurance committee.

First, no performance data or information exist on how well, or even how many, cardiopulmonary resuscitations are being performed in the hospital. The extent of knowledge about these resuscitations consists of notes in some of the affected patients' records, charges billed for items such as medications used during resuscitations, and knowledge of one medical liability suit recently filed after an unsuccessful resuscitation. Second, neither a performance measurement system nor performance measures exist to provide quantitative performance data and information about this process of care or its outcomes.

Third, there is no dependable mechanism for teaching CPR to house staff members, medical staff, nurses, and other health professionals who participate in cardiopulmonary resuscitations. A cursory survey of medical staff reveals one individual qualified to teach the American Heart Association's advanced cardiac life support (ACLS) resuscitation guidelines.[1] Some nurses, house staff members, and medical staff who work in the hospital's special care and emergency units have been trained in ACLS elsewhere. They now restrict their participation in cardiac resuscitations to those occurring within their units.

Fourth, house staff members are not supervised by medical staff during cardiopulmonary resuscitations. Fifth, there are no written guidelines as to how CPR should be performed in the hospital. Most of the physicians and other providers participating in CPR use their best judgment as to what medication should be used for a given dysrhythmia or when to perform endotracheal intubation. The task force members remark that it is impossible to measure compliance with guidelines when written performance guidelines outlining expectations do not exist. Sixth, some of the equipment available to perform cardiopulmonary resuscitations is old, ineffective, and unsafe. The oxygen tubing in the cardiopulmonary kits, for instance, is incompatible with the oxygen outlets in various parts of the hospital.

The task force makes several recommendations. First, written guidelines regarding performance of CPR should be developed, adopted, or adapted from existing guidelines. Second, all resuscitations performed by house staff members should be supervised by medical staff. If an attending physician is not physically present at the resuscitation, responsibility lies with the house staff member conducting the resuscitation to report the procedure to an attending physician.

Third, performance data from each resuscitation should be collected and analyzed. The data specifically should include a description of the key decisions taken during the resuscitation, immediate outcome of the resuscitation, and whether the patient survives to discharge from the hospital. Administration is asked to provide funds to support a part-time individual to collect these data. Fourth, old equipment should be replaced and new equipment added to the cardiopulmonary resuscitation carts. Fifth, basic cardiac life support (BCLS) should be offered to all employees who desire it.

One year later work continues on taking action on these recommendations. The certified ACLS physician instructor, for example, suggests that ACLS emergency cardiac care guidelines should be adopted and taught to staff members rather than using scarce organizational resources to create a second set of guidelines. Some medical staff, however, believe that they can develop superior guidelines and resist a "cookbook approach" to providing emergency cardiac care. Many medical staff have not had time to read the American Heart Association's guidelines.

Representatives of administration state that money is scarce and funding of the part-time individual to collect resuscitation data must come from a department's existing budget. The department heads disagree on who should assume this responsibility. A subcommittee is formed to investigate the purchase of adaptors so that oxygen tubing will be compatible with oxygen outlets throughout the hospital, but the committee, composed mostly of physicians, is having difficulty finding time to meet and does not know whom to contact about oxygen tubing. The hospital administration expresses disappointment with numerous clinical units and the hospital quality assurance committee when the hospital accreditation report cites serious deficiencies throughout the organization, including lack of compliance with standards relating to CPR.

There are several important lessons to be gleaned from this hospital's experience. First, the complexity of patient care should never be underestimated. Beyond the clinical care provided directly to the patient, governance decisions, management oversight and coordination, and adequacy of support services all factor into the health outcomes realized by patients. Multiple participants often become involved, directly or indirectly, in the care process. This involvement becomes increasingly complex when the patient's illness or injury is serious.

In this example, the CPR committee uncovered not one, but several, interlinked performance areas that needed improvement, including provider education; information management; leadership; performance assessment and improvement; and plant, technology, and safety management. One lesson learned was that the large number of opportunities to improve CPR should have signaled organizational leadership to assume responsibility for organizing and fostering the efforts of individuals and groups needed for ongoing performance measurement, assessment, and improvement of the hospital's CPR system. Leadership not only failed to meet this need, but it also blamed the individuals and units whose performance it believed led to an undesirable hospital survey accreditation outcome.

A second lesson learned from this hospital's experience is that internally driven improvement efforts are more likely to result in lasting and substantive improvements than externally driven improvement efforts such as external inspection processes, patient complaints, or medical liability suits.

A growing number of organizations, especially those that have adopted a version of the continuous improvement paradigm described in detail elsewhere, have a heightened awareness of their need to survive in the current health care environment.[3-5] They recognize their own complexity and fragility and are driven to do as well as they can in providing care. They understand that this desire must be in large part internally driven and cannot be externally imposed. Indeed, many organizations are beginning to understand that improvement efforts are most likely to be effective when internal and external sources of motivation operate in concert rather than in opposition or not at all.

The excellent clinical performance improvement opportunity identified by two conscientious, patient-focused providers in this example was unfortunately doomed to failure as the project was effectively moved from patients' bedsides into the domain of a hospital committee. There the modus operandi shifted away from meeting the needs of patients to meeting the immediate needs of the organization, which at the time were to maintain its hospital accreditation status.

Leadership did not grasp the important link between how well an organization conducts performance measurement and improvement and its ability to thrive in an environment (purchasers, patients, accreditors) demanding excellence in performance. Leadership failed to understand that improved performance is inherently desirable for the organization. Health care organizations that take charge of their own performance issues are those most likely to survive and thrive in the current era of public accountability. These organizations are likely to exceed external review requirements as a simple by-product of their own efforts.

A third lesson learned from this hospital's experience is that performance measurement, assessment, and improvement are not simply paper-shuffling exercises to be performed just prior to an accreditation survey. Instead, health care organizations must continuously weave performance measurement and improvement processes into their day-to-day activities. Organizations that are successful in achieving these goals will be able to demonstrate to patients, payers, accrediting bodies, and other groups their actual level of performance in providing the services they are supposed to be capable of delivering.

A fourth lesson learned from this hospital's experience is that performance measurement and improvement efforts become less effective when ignorance, arrogance, and turf battles are allowed to interfere with improvement projects. In this example, the organization and its units cannot even *begin* the measurement process because they cannot agree on who is going to pay for the measurer or whose measurement guidelines and instruments will be used. The likelihood of collecting and analyzing performance data, and using analyses to identify opportunities to improve the care of patients, correlates directly with the extent to which individuals, units, and organizations allow themselves to be subject to expected organizational behaviors. Management philosophies, such as total quality management and continuous quality improvement, offer promise in reducing ignorance and arrogance by focusing the organization's energies on meeting the needs of its customers.

CASE 2: Performance Measurement and the "Halo Effect"

Hospital B provides emergency services to more than a thousand trauma patients per year of which approximately half have sustained penetrating (for instance, stab wounds, gunshot wounds) injuries and the other half blunt (for instance, motor vehicle accidents, falls) injuries.

Responsibility for the care of trauma patients in the emergency unit is shared between surgical and emergency medicine house staff members who are "covered" by attending physicians who can be reached by telephone or beeper when they are not physically present in the emergency unit. A senior surgical house staff member is responsible for performing all primary surgical evaluations in the emergency unit for a given 24-hour period. This is his or her chief responsibility for a one-month period, although he or she may participate in surgical procedures and other activities elsewhere in the hospital when the emergency unit does not require his or her services.

The senior surgical house staff member carries a beeper when he or she is not physically present in the emergency unit for notification of the impending or actual arrival of trauma patients. Emergency medicine house staff members and attending physicians are responsible for providing care to all trauma and nontrauma patients who present to the emergency unit.

An opportunity to improve the timeliness with which surgical house staff members respond after being paged for trauma patients is suggested by emergency medicine house staff members. They decide to measure the performance timeliness of the surgical house staff members—that is, the degree to which services, procedures, tests, and treatments are provided by these physicians when they are needed by trauma patients—for several weeks. The unit of measure selected is minutes. The indicator is the minutes elapsed between the time the surgical house staff member is notified of impending (or actual) trauma patient arrival and the time he or she first responds to the notification.

A trauma response survey form is designed (see Figure 18) and completed by emergency medicine house staff for 35 of 70 consecutive trauma cases (every other case) during a three-week measurement period. The data shown in Table 11 are divided into two periods. Surgical house staff members are unaware of the monitoring during the first data collection period and have become aware of the monitoring during the second data collection period.

During the first week of the performance measurement period the mean response time is 54 minutes with a range of 15 to 165 minutes. During the second and third weeks of measurement, the mean response is 8 minutes with a range of 0 to 155 minutes. When two response times are deleted from the data set (in each instance the paging or pager system was not working), the mean response time is less than one minute during the second and third weeks of measurement.

The marked improvement of surgical house staff members' response time as illustrated by a comparison of the two data analysis periods is attributed to the "halo effect" by those familiar with the measurement project. This means that improvement in performance occurs when individuals, departments, and/or disciplines become aware that their performance is being measured.

Figure 18

Trauma Response Survey Form*

Date ___ *mm/dd/yy* _____   Shift: 7–3   3–11   <u>11–7</u>

Trauma Log # ___ *xx* _____

Case Description: ___ *Patient in high-speed motor vehicle* _____

___ *accident; decreased mental status with ?* _____

___ *history of head trauma and loss of* _____

___ *consciousness. Smells of alcohol.* _____

___ *Vital signs stable. Blood in urine.* _____

___ *2330* ___   Time emergency unit staff member notified of patient arrival (if applicable)

___ *2340* ___   Time senior surgical resident first paged

___ *0215* ___   First response any surgical resident

___ *0215* ___   First response senior surgical resident

___ *Several* ___   *Repeat pages, telephone, four bells*

Issues

___ *xx* ___   No response for __ *155* __ minutes

_____   Paged out

___ *xx* ___   In surgery

_____   Confusion (for example, Who is on call? versus Who is listed on the oncall list?)

___ *xx* ___   Other ___ *Resident states that pager system down* _____

_____

Comments ___ *Neurosurgery resident physician successfully paged* _____

___ *at 2345 and arrived at 0015.* _____

* Data are hypothetical.

Table 11

Trauma Response Time Data*

Data Collected First Week		Data Collected Second and Third Week	
Case #	Response Time (minutes)	Case #	Response Time (minutes)
1	165	9	3 minutes
2	15	10	0†
3	35	11	155
4	25	12	5
5	65	13	0†
6	25	14	0†
7	20	15	0†
8	85	16	0†
		17	50
Total: 435		18	2
		19	0†
Mean: 54 minutes		20	0
Range: 15-165 minutes		21	1
		22	3
		23	0†
		24	0†
		25	1
		26	3
		27	0†
		28	0†
		29	2
		30	0†
		31	0†
		32	0†
		33	0†
		34	3
		35	0†
		Total:	228
		Mean:	8.1 minutes
		Range:	0-155 minutes

*These data are hypothetical.

†Senior surgical house staff member present in the emergency unit.

The halo effect is often transitory and can disappear when individuals, departments, and/or disciplines believe that performance measurement has ceased. There are at least two approaches to maintaining a higher level of performance: Measurement must continue, or the system should be redesigned.

In Hospital B, resources (emergency unit staff members' time and other resources) are insufficient to support ongoing quantification of the timeliness with which surgical house staff members respond after being paged for trauma patients. The improved performance achieved through the halo effect is sustained nevertheless by improving communication, awareness, and respect between surgical and emergency medicine attending staff members and house staff members who become closely involved with continuously studying and improving the care of trauma patients. In the absence of continuous performance measurement, it is difficult to ascertain how long the relatively high level of performance will last, however—especially in the face of heavy and rapid staff member turnover.

CASE 3: Potential Results of Performance Measurement When Organizational Leadership and an Individual Unit Have Different Objectives

Hospital C provides emergency services for approximately 45,000 patients per year. Of these 45,000 patients, 20%, or 9,000, are admitted as inpatients to the hospital. Emergency medicine staff members perceive a potential opportunity to improve the timeliness with which patients are admitted from the emergency unit to the hospital. There is a perception that the admission process is long and is one factor contributing to overcrowding in the emergency unit and possibly to poor outcomes in some patients.

A multiple-week study is conducted by emergency unit staff members to collect performance data to determine the timeliness with which the admission process is performed. Specific times are recorded by emergency unit staff members on the Admission Process Survey Form depicted in Figure 19. Five time periods are measured:

Period 1: Time admission slip is submitted to the emergency unit clerk to the time admission is entered into the computer;

Period 2: Time admission is entered into computer by the clerk to the time a bed is assigned by admissions office personnel;

Period 3: Time the bed is assigned to the time the bed is ready;

Period 4: Time the bed is ready to the time the patient leaves the emergency unit; and

Period 5: Time the admission slip is submitted to the emergency unit clerk to the time the patient leaves the emergency unit (the sum of periods 1 through 4).

Figure 19
Admission Process Survey Form

Admitting Service _____

Type of Bed: _____ICU   _____Monitored   _____Isolation   _____Floor

_____ Time admit slip submitted (physician/clerk)

_____ Time entered into computer (clerk)

_____ Time bed is assigned (clerk)

_____ Time bed is ready (clerk)

_____ Time patient leaves Emergency Department (nurse/physician)

Problems

_____No beds in hospital

_____Bed not clean

_____Admitting not aware of bed request

_____Bed not empty yet; no other bed available

_____Bed not empty yet; other empty beds available

_____Nurses in report

_____Bed assigned, but Emergency Department not notified

_____Service-specified bed not available

_____Other, explain: _____

The means and ranges for data collected for periods 1 through 5 are the following:

Period 1: 7 minutes (mean), 0-50 minutes (range);
Period 2: 78 minutes (mean), 0-345 minutes (range);
Period 3: 26 minutes (mean), 0-190 minutes (range);
Period 4: 30 minutes (mean), 0-310 minutes (range); and
Period 5: 133 minutes (mean), 0-660 minutes (range).

In 63 of the 171 cases, an underlying problem is identified by emergency unit staff members. These problems include bed not clean (20 cases); bed assigned but emergency unit not notified (11 cases); no bed available in the hospital (11 cases); admitting service resident physicians conducting additional patient evaluation in the emergency unit (10 cases); bed to which patient assigned not yet empty (8 cases); admission office clerk not notifying receiving ward (2 cases); and admission office clerk is not aware of bed request (1 case).

Emergency unit staff members request an appointment with admissions office staff members to communicate their findings and try to find ways to improve the timeliness with which the admissions function is carried out in the hospital. The admissions office staff members and administration are anxious to meet with emergency unit staff members about separate concerns.

The major concern of hospital administration and the admissions office is the increasing number of self-pay and Medicaid patients who are being admitted to the hospital through the emergency unit. The timeliness with which these and other patients are admitted to the hospital through the emergency unit is a lesser priority.

Hospital leadership subsequently focuses admission function improvement efforts on reducing the number of self-pay/Medicaid patients admitted to the hospital through the emergency unit by fostering transfer of such patients from the emergency unit to other institutions after preliminary assessment. This, in theory, will free up hospital beds, they reason, and improve the timeliness with which other (paying) patients will be admitted.

This solution does not address the crowding issue in the emergency unit or the issue of patient dumping. No other action is taken on the performance data collected during the performance measurement study conducted by emergency unit staff members.

There are several important lessons to learn from this vignette. First, this case study again shows the enormous complexity of patient care demonstrated in the first case study. Admission to a given hospital today involves more than needing to be hospitalized, giving consent, signing a few forms, and being wheeled to a bed. House staff members may detain patients in the emergency department for evaluation and additional diagnostic workup, housekeeping may be busy elsewhere, nurses may be changing shifts, and/or hospital procedures and policies may direct the placement of patients elsewhere whose ability to pay for services cannot be ensured.

A second lesson relating to this hospital's experience is that a single organizational unit—however well-intentioned—is unlikely to correct a multidepartmental, multidisciplinary problem such as the timeliness with which patients are admitted to the hospital. The admissions function crosses multiple departmental and disciplinary boundaries, and each department and discipline is likely to have its own perspective on the admissions process. Measurement and improvement of the admissions function should be organized, supported, and fostered by the organization's leadership.

A third lesson learned from this hospital's experience is that leadership usually prevails over individuals and units of the organization, even when the motives and actions of leadership may not support the best interests of patients or providers.

CASE 4: Potential Impact of Data Quality on Performance Measurement

Hospital D joins a regional trauma network that requires collection of basic data elements about each trauma patient evaluated by, and admitted to, the hospital. These data include, for instance, Glasgow Coma Score (a measure of severity of injury), mechanism of injury, number of days hospitalized, frequency of operative procedures, mortality, and payer status. Trauma patient records are removed from the emergency unit and abstracted during night shifts by hospital-based radio dispatchers located elsewhere in the hospital.

The purpose of data collection is to build a regional trauma care database and to monitor the quality and quantity of care provided by individual hospitals within the trauma network. Each month for 12 months, Hospital D sends its trauma "statistics" to the regional headquarters for inclusion in the regional database (see Table 12). Employment of a new hospital chief executive officer, a new surgery director, and a new emergency unit director has precluded the review of these data prior to their submission.

The new surgery and emergency unit directors review the aggregate regional trauma data one day noting that Hospital D's monthly count of trauma cases appears to be low compared to other hospitals in the area and low in comparison to their subjective recountings. The directors organize a review of the data collection process to ascertain the degree to which the data being submitted by Hospital D to the regional database are reliable.

The first challenge is to find the individual who can and will retrieve all of the trauma data from the hospital computer where they are stored. When this is eventually accomplished, the data are analyzed for their degrees of completeness and accuracy. Data completeness is measured by reabstracting all emergency unit trauma patient records for two recent months and comparing the data in each record to the corresponding data in Hospital D's trauma database. There is difficulty in locating some trauma patient emergency unit

Table 12

Trauma Statistics Report by Glasgow Coma Score
Month of January, 19xx*

Glasgow Coma Scores					Total #	Hospital
<7	7–9	10–12	13–14	15	Patients	Identification
0	0	4	4	42	50	Hospital A
0	0	0	1	34	35	Hospital B
1	0	1	3	6	11	Hospital C
3	0	3	1	30	37	**Hospital D**
0	0	2	8	81	91	Hospital E
3	6	35	26	184	254	Hospital F
0	0	2	3	70	75	Hospital G
0	1	2	1	76	80	Hospital H

*These data are hypothetical.

records because they are in various parts of the hospital or have been lost. Reabstracting the patient records that can be found reveals two findings that seriously threaten data quality and undermine the degree to which the data can be trusted by users.

First, the database contains many types of inaccuracies or errors. The database, for instance, contains data derived from *nontraumatic* resuscitations performed in the emergency unit involving, for instance, patients with nontraumatic cardiac arrest, severe gastrointestinal bleeding, sepsis, bradycardia, and nontraumatic subarachnoid hemorrhage (see Table 13). The database also contains a prehospital Glasgow Coma Score for each patient even though prehospital records containing this information cannot be located for most of the trauma patients. The Glasgow Coma Score and the measurements from which it can be derived are not consistently documented by providers in the emergency unit trauma patient record. This eliminates the possibility that the abstractors derived the Glasgow Coma Score from the emergency unit patient record.

Second, the database is incomplete. Reviewers find that data derived from care of *more than half* of all the trauma patients evaluated in the emergency unit and admitted to the hospital are *not* contained in Hospital D's database. This finding confirms the directors' initial sense that the number of trauma patients cared for by Hospital D staff members is not accurately reflected in the regional trauma database statistics.

The unit directors bring their conclusions to the attention of individuals responsible for data abstraction and the data collection process. There are many reasons why the data are not perfect, they say, including inability of staff members to locate patient records, illegible handwriting on patient records, inadequate resources, inadequate training, human error, lack of commitment to the measurement process, and lack of an ongoing review process to determine the reliability of the data. Data collection is interrupted while the issue is being considered. Staff members at the regional trauma database headquarters make inquiries several months later as to why no statistics are being submitted by Hospital D.

The major lesson taught by this case study is that the quality of performance data is one of the most important issues in any performance measurement system because a wide range of organization

Table 13

Data Inaccuracy Due to Nontrauma Cases
Entered into Hospital D's Trauma Database*

Case Number	Type of Medical Illness
231	Cardiac arrest
249	Cardiac arrest
256	Cardiac arrest
257	Cardiac arrest
258	Medical hypotension
259	Cardiac arrest
267	Cardiac arrest
268	Cardiac arrest
271	Cerebral vascular accident
278	Chest pain/hypertension
285	Cardiac arrest
290	Drug overdose
294	Seizures/hypotension
296	No data at all
318	Pulmonary embolus
331	Cardiac arrest
344	Cardiac arrest
345	Subarachnoid hemorrhage
346	Sepsis
357	Bradycardia
359	Gastrointestinal bleeding
369	Cardiac arrest
380	Cardiac arrest
385	Pulmonary edema
401	Gastrointestinal bleeding
411	Drug ingestion
414	Drug ingestion
416	Cardiac arrest
417	Cardiac arrest
419	Cardiac arrest
426	Cardiac arrest
430	Cardiac arrest
452	Cardiac arrest
463	Cardiac arrest
466	Cardiac arrest
473	Ventricular fibrillation
478	Cardiac arrest
481	Cardiac arrest
486	Cardiac arrest
503	Cardiac arrest
519	Cardiac arrest
522	Ventricular tachycardia
534	Heat stroke

*These data are hypothetical.

activities may be triggered as a result of these data. Grossly inaccurate and incomplete data such as those collected and submitted by Hospital D can contaminate a regional database, rendering statistical analyses, such as calculation of group means and standard deviations, meaningless or misleading not only to Hospital D but to all the hospitals contributing to the database.

The potential for contaminated databases is one reason why the Joint Commission has devoted considerable resources to developing, testing, revising, and then retesting computer software and manual abstraction tools for the beta phase of indicator testing. This approach increases the probability that accurate and complete data elements are abstracted and submitted by health care organizations to the Joint Commission database (see Chapter Seven). The collection and submission of unreliable data, which foul databases and render them less useful and misleading to users, represent a reprehensible and indefensible waste of health care resources.

Summary Observations

The process of measuring or quantifying performance of everyday processes and the outcomes achieved can present many challenges to organizations. Some of these challenges have been described in this chapter and are summarized as follows.

1. Organizations should be prepared for discovering and dealing with multiple interlinked issues when a substantive multidisciplinary and multidepartmental project, such as improving cardiopulmonary resuscitation services, is initially identified.

2. Performance measurement will more likely result in performance improvement when it is internally, rather than externally, driven. Organizations that foster performance measurement for the sake of continuously improving services provided to patients, payers, and other users are likely to exceed any external review requirements that may be set.

3. Ignorance, arrogance, and interdepartmental/interdisciplinary posturing will threaten the success of improvement projects. This is why it is important for organizational leadership to consider embracing management philosophies, such as total quality management or continuous quality improvement, that recognize and effectively deal with these human conditions.

4. The halo effect is the transitory improvement in performance that results solely from awareness that measurement of performance is taking place.

5. A single department or discipline—however well-intentioned—is unlikely to successfully improve an organizationwide systemic problem.

6. Organizational leadership is likely to prevail in areas where its objectives conflict with those of an individual unit within the organization.

7. The quality of performance data submitted to a database is an important consideration in judging the trustworthiness and validity of any measurement derived from the database. The quality of performance data is also important because of the wide range of activities that may be triggered as a result of that data. Data quality can be threatened by many factors ranging from lack of commitment to illegible handwriting.

References

1. American Heart Association. Guidelines for cardiopulmonary resuscitation and emergency cardiac care. 1992. *JAMA* 268:2172–2302.

2. Joint Commission on Accreditation of Healthcare Organizations. 1988. *Accreditation Manual for Hospitals, 1989 Edition, Volume I.* Oakbrook Terrace, IL, pp 38,58,140,141,187,236,238,272.

3. Joint Commission on Accreditation of Healthcare Organizations. 1991. *An Introduction to Quality Improvement in Healthcare.* Oakbrook Terrace, IL.

4. Kritchevsky SB, Simmons BP. 1991. Continuous quality improvement. *JAMA* 266:1817–1823.

5. Berwick DF. 1989. Continuous improvement as an ideal in health care. *N Engl J Med* 320:53–56.

A

The Minimum Standard*

1. That physicians and surgeons privileged to practice in the hospital be organized as a definite group or staff. Such organization has nothing to do with the question as to whether the hospital is "open" or "closed," nor need it affect the various existing types of staff organization. The word STAFF is here defined as the group of doctors who practice in the hospital inclusive of all groups such as the "regular staff," "the visiting staff," and the "associate staff."

2. That membership upon the staff be restricted to physicians and surgeons who are (a) full graduates of medicine in good standing and legally licensed to practice in their respective states or provinces, (b) competent in their respective fields, and (c) worthy in character and in matters of professional ethics; that in this latter connection the practice of the division of fees, under any guise whatever, be prohibited.

3. That the staff initiate and, with the approval of the governing board of the hospital, adopt rules, regulations, and policies governing the professional work of the hospital: that these rules, regulations, and policies specifically provide:

(a) That staff meetings be held at least once each month. (In large hospitals the departments may choose to meet separately.)

(b) That the staff review and analyze at regular intervals their clinical experience in the various departments of the hospital, such as medicine, surgery, obstetrics, and the other specialties; the clinical

---

*Adopted in 1919 by the American College of Surgeons for use in its Hospital Standardization Program.

records of patients, free and pay, to be the basis for such review and analyses.

4. That accurate and complete records be written for all patients and filed in an accessible manner in the hospital—a complete case record being one which includes identification data; complaint; personal and family history; history of present illness; physical examination, special examinations, such as consultations, clinical laboratory, X-ray and other examinations; provisional or working diagnosis; medical or surgical treatment; gross and microscopical pathological findings; progress notes; final diagnosis; condition on discharge; follow-up and, in case of death, autopsy findings.

5. That diagnostic and therapeutic facilities under competent supervision be available for the study, diagnosis, and treatment of patients, these to include, at least (a) a clinical laboratory providing chemical, bacteriological, serological, and pathological services, (b) an X-ray department providing radiographic and fluoroscopic services.

B

Transcript of "The Medical Audit" by Paul S. Ferguson, MD, Acting Assistant Director, American College of Surgeons, in Charge of Hospital Activities, Circa Early 1950s*

In the business end of hospital management it is considered essential to have systematic audits made of the books in which income and outgo of funds are recorded. When the auditors make their reports the administrator and board members spend considerable time studying the results, analyzing them and discussing what can be done to improve the financial position of the hospital.

This is as it should be. Patients benefit when hospitals are well managed from a business standpoint; nevertheless, this is an incidental consideration compared with good management from a professional standpoint. The patient entrusts his life to the hospital and the people who serve in it. Surely an audit of the records of his and his fellow patients' reactions to treatment is infinitely more important than an audit of cash receipts and expenditures. The primary concern of the hospital should be a good balance sheet in terms of progress in saving lives. Yet, how few hospitals, comparatively speaking, make thorough medical audits as systematically as they do financial audits!

Of course, after a fashion, some analyses of the clinical results have been made in most hospitals for a long time. The term "medical audit" is rather new, but the principle is not. Actually, whenever a medical staff meets to analyze the clinical work of the hospital a sort of medical audit takes place. Ever since it started Hospital Standardization in 1918 the American College of Surgeons has stressed the holding of regular monthly medical staff conferences at which a

---

*Source: Joint Commission Archives, Oakbrook Terrace, IL.

thorough review of the clinical work should take place. Recently, however, hospital administrators, medical staffs and governing boards have come to think of the medical audit in a more formal sense because of the promotion of this idea by the College.

The medical audit is a stimulus to the practice of scientific medicine. It is an objective and specific check on the professional work performed in the hospital. It is an account of the medical care rendered in terms of lives saved, avoidable and unavoidable deaths, diseases arrested, and patients rehabilitated and restored to a society as healthy, happy, productive people. In the last analysis, the medical audit informs the governing board of the work of each physician on the staff and places it (The Board) in a favorable position to judge the competency or incompetency of the members of the medical staff.

The medical audit is carried on with varying degrees of thoroughness and value. It is estimated that approximately 150,000 medical staff conferences are held each year in the United States to review and analyze the clinical work of the hospital.

Dr Henry G. Farish, in his article in the July, 1949 issue of "Modern Hospital," states that the hospital can be assured the work of its medical staff is reasonably efficient in two ways:

1. It can set up a system of professional accounting upon which a medical audit can be done at periodic intervals.

2. It may engage a qualified physician, independent of the medical staff, to scrutinize in detail the results of the medical work of the hospital over a specified period of time.

A good medical audit considers some ten basic factors of good medical care. Some are more evident than others, but all are important facets of patient care and must be considered if the objectives are to be accomplished.

1. *The average bed occupancy.* It may seem strange to bring bed occupancy into the discussion, but there is good reason for doing so. There seems to be uniform agreement that an 80% occupancy is the top limit for safety and efficient care. A higher rate of occupancy may render the services performed by the medical, nursing, and non-professional staffs less effective due to pressure of work, limited space, and over-use of facilities and supplies. Overcrowding reduces the amount of oxygen available and creates the danger of exposure to infections, as well as increasing the difficulty of providing adequate

care needed by the patient. Such conditions are reflected in the progress of the patient. A longer convalescence may result, perhaps marked by complications, due to the physical handicaps which surround the patient and set up barriers to good patient care. It is surprising, however, to note that our hospitals in recent years have maintained a generally high standard despite overcrowding. Good techniques, coupled with advances in chemotherapy, must receive a large share of the credit for this result.

2. *Average days' stay.* In a medical audit we must consider the average days' stay since this so often reflects the quality of medical care. It is true that since 1918, the year in which Hospital Standardization originated, the average days' stay of patients in acute hospitals has dropped dramatically. Not too long ago the average days' stay in the hospital was 24 to 26 days or even higher. This has dropped to an average of 6 to 10 days. The reduction can be attributed to scientific medical care, better nursing, and to a certain extent the principle of early ambulation. The progress of medical science has in turn stimulated the initiation of more efficient organization and administration of hospitals, the development and expansion of the adjunct facilities of the hospital, intern and resident training programs, medical staff conferences, and all the other elements operative under the Hospital Standardization Program. These have produced notable results.

Today an average stay of 15 or more days is indicative of need for investigation and study. This could denote several significant factors: (1) care of chronic and incurable patients in a hospital intended for acute patients; (2) poor medical care resulting in complications and untoward sequelae; (3) dilatory care by the individual physician. It has often been noted that some physicians see their patients daily while they are in the hospital, and do everything possible to speed their recovery. Other physicians seem to forget about their patients, fail to visit them until reminded to do so, and wait a long period of time for the patient to improve without seeking the benefit of medical consultation. In fact, it would be well for the hospital to record the average days' stay of the patients on each service, because this will show in an indirect way the quality of medical care given patients by individual physicians. It is also well to approach the length of hospital stay on the basis of diagnosis. This variation by physicians is an important factor to investigate. Generally there is a reason for the variation, one more or less directly associated with the temperament, the competency, and probably the interest of the individual physician.

3. *Gross Results.* The gross results of patient care in a specified period of time point up the areas which need to be given more careful analysis. The figures covering the number of patients recovered, improved, not treated, in for diagnosis, and died are significant of the over-all patient care given in the institution, and should be reviewed carefully.

4. *The Death Rate.* The death rate as a whole and on the various services may be a good indication of the proficiency of the medical care. The present average of 3% to 4% (in some cases much lower) should be used as a basic criterion with such exceptions as are necessary for city and county hospitals or other institutions which receive a great many moribund cases. It is well to record both the general death rate of the hospital and the rate of each of the services, taking into consideration reasonable modifying factors.

A postoperative death rate of more than 1% is considered outside the bounds of normal limits unless extenuating circumstances are present. The existing low average rate is indicative of the advance in surgical skill. A contributing factor is the improvement in anesthesia equipment and technique. Competent physician anesthetists in charge of skilled nurse anesthetists have helped to reduce surgical risks to a minimum. Today not more than one death in every 5,000 operations should be attributed to anesthesia.

A drop in the maternal and infant death rate over the past 15 to 50 years has been dramatic. Today a maternal death rate of more than .25% and an infant death rate of more than 2% is considered high and is, or should be, immediately investigated by city or county authorities as well as by the medical staff.

5. *Consultations.* As a result of the hospital surveys conducted over many years as a part of the approval program of the American College of Surgeons, the conclusion has been reached that formal consultations could be held to advantage on 15% to 20% of all patients entering a general hospital. It is believed that the general results in the hospital follow pretty much the curve of incidence of consultations. This does not mean the informal consultation, the one held in the

corridor, the doctors' room, or on the parking lot. A formal consultation must be held at the bedside, the history studied, an examination must be carefully made by the consultant and the findings recorded after a discussion between the attending physician and the consultant or consultants. The rules and regulations of the medical staff should stipulate the type of cases in which consultations are mandatory. Generally these are required in cases of therapeutic abortion and sterilization. There is no question whatsoever that a higher grade of medical service will be found in the hospital recording a high percentage of formal consultations.

6. *Infections.* The incidence of infection is a particularly valuable index in judging the surgical and obstetrical services. A ratio of more than 1 $1/2$% to 2% of infections, postoperatively, in clean surgical cases calls for investigation. A similar plan should be applied to maternal care, although infections in maternity cases are now very well regulated by the morbidity standard promulgated by the American Committee on Maternal Welfare. In clean surgery followed by infection, there is always a definite cause which can be found and against which preventive measures can be enforced.

Investigations have unearthed a number of startling reasons for the occurrence of infections. There was the horseback rider enthusiast who, after his invigorating early morning canter, came to the operating floor in a riding habit. After a hasty shower and a rapid change of clothing he prepared to operate. A break in the technique of sterilizing the hands caused three cases of tetanus followed by two deaths. It is obvious that the source of infection could definitely be traced to the surgeon.

An incidence of 16$2/3$% infections of clean surgical cases in a large surgical ward revealed that the intern assigned to the floor was not following the correct technical procedure in dressing wounds. As he went from patient to patient, he dipped the instruments in a common Lysol solution and did not wash his hands between patients.

In another hospital showing a great many postoperative infections, a survey revealed twenty-one breaks in the operating room technique, all of which were remediable.

These stories emphasize the need for alertness and investigation of all infections in any hospital, particularly in those institutions in which a high incidence of infections occurs. Generally the cause can be found and proper prevention and control instituted.

7. *Complications following clean surgical cases, obstetrical cases, and medical cases.* All such complications may be prevented in large measure and should not occur more frequently than in 3% to 4% of the cases. The postoperative pneumonia or the postoperative bronchitis may be due to quite apparent causes and should not occur with any degree of frequency. It is true that we cannot prevent some complications, such as embolism, and thrombosis of the veins of the extremities following operation, but we can check techniques and see that infective processes are kept to the lowest minimum. Complications usually indicate a weakness somewhere in the service. They should be studied and preventive measures instituted.

8. *Unnecessary surgery.* The frequency of certain operations may lead to a suspicion that operations are being performed which are not based on legitimate diagnoses. We find in many hospitals that a large number of appendectomies and hysterectomies are performed. Perhaps the most alarming incidence of this type is the increase in the number of cesarean sections. Such cases should never be higher than 3% to 4% with a possible outer limit of 5%. A higher percentage calls for investigation and the institution of preventive measures, such as a carefully recorded history, pelvic measurements, and formal consultations. There seems to be a growing tendency to perform cesarean sections and sterilizations upon the request of the patient. This should never be permitted. Such procedures should be carried out only when the life of the mother or the baby is at stake, or to promote the future health of the mother if she is suffering from an accompanying disease, such as tuberculosis, a heart condition, arthritis, or the like. Operations should never be performed without written indications that justify the procedure.

9. *Autopsy rate.* Great stress is laid on the incidence of autopsies. Generally these should not be less than 20% to 30% in the average hospital although there are justifiable reasons for a lesser percentage. In certain hospitals where there are only private patients the autopsy rate may be lower than in a county or city hospital although frequently the reverse is true. It is always well for the hospital to have a record of the general incidence of autopsies broken down as to services. Naturally this will vary. The dermatologist, the otolaryngologist, and the ophthalmologist will rate much lower than the pediatrician, the general surgeon or the urologist. Therefore, due

consideration must be given to the service and not infrequently to the type of patient.

It is truly said that the incidence of autopsies is a good indication of the scientific interest of the medical staff; therefore this index should be carefully watched and should come under the scrutiny of the medical staff or the person responsible for the audit.

10. *Staff conferences.* The quality of patient care and the scientific spirit of the members of the medical staff is in direct proportion to the number of medical staff conferences held routinely for the analysis of clinical work. These include general medical staff meetings, departmental staff conferences, and clinicopathology conferences. The group spirit and scientific attitude demonstrated in these conferences enhance the role of the physician and promote safe and proficient care of the patient. Great stress should be laid on productive conferences of this nature; in fact it may be said that a scientific atmosphere cannot prevail in a hospital which lacks adequate medical conferences, and that a medical staff unable to cooperate to the extent necessary to produce such meetings fails to warrant the confidence of the governing board of the hospital. It is the duty, the responsibility, and the obligation not only of the medical staff but of the administrator and the board of trustees to cooperate in providing the best possible care to the patient in order to return him as quickly as possible to his place in society.

The foregoing ten factors of good medical care are obviously basic. Probably you would be interested in the reasoning which has led to the increasing emphasis upon the medical audit. Many of you knew the late Dr Thomas R. Ponton who for many years was associated directly and indirectly with the College in its Hospital Standardization Program. Doctor Ponton was perhaps the earliest proponent of the professional audit idea. He made the following explanation of his interest in a talk in 1939 at the Clinical Congress of the American College of Surgeons:

"Because of the lack of effective methods of staff control, the possibility of determining competence from actual records of performance had been a matter of interest to me since the beginning of my hospital experience. In every hospital in which I was engaged as superintendent or consultant, I kept a private record of the work of the individual members of the medical staff. I was particularly concerned about devising some method which would provide safeguards against the deterioration which may result when an older physician does not keep up with the advances that are constantly taking place in the practice of medicine—safeguards which are equally as important as those we know should be set up against the inexperienced younger surgeon. I gradually developed a system which in 1929 had become sufficiently practical to warrant presentation at a meeting of this organization (The ACS) in a paper entitled "Measuring the Work of the Physician." Encouraged by the reception of the idea, I went ahead and further developed the system of professional accounting and added the idea of a professional audit. The essential point of professional accounting is that, for each patient, there must be an honest comparison of the result secured with those which may be reasonably expected. This comparison must be made by a competent medical authority and any criticism which may result must be constructive in character. The objective is not to place blame on any individual or on the hospital organization and routine, but rather to find successes and failures of all kinds in order to bring out a constant improvement in the work of the hospital organization, of the medical staff as a whole, and of the individual staff members."

Doctor Ponton in his promotion of the idea of professional audits stressed the importance of good medical statistics, and we make the same emphasis today. Well trained and capable medical record librarians and statisticians were never more needed than they are now when we recognize their function in contributing to good medical auditing. Also the medical staff members must be medical records conscious. Again we draw a parallel between the medical and the financial balance sheet—there could be no true financial audit if every transaction were not entered—neither can there be a true medical audit if every symptom, procedure, reaction, observation and result is not conscientiously and promptly recorded. The quality of the medical record in itself is one of the first subjects for appraisal in the medical audit. A medical audit does not necessarily uncover altogether unpleasant facts. In many instances the reverse is true. It may disclose accomplishments beyond average. It is just as important that we know in what direction good results are being achieved as it is that we know wherein we are deficient.

A Michigan hospital administrator recently reported to us that the institution of a medical audit in his hospital had produced some agreeable surprises. Rumors had spread in his community that many unnecessary operations were being performed. These rumors had been growing so persistent and loud that the doctors themselves began to share the feeling, each suspecting the others. An unhappy atmosphere had begun to pervade the hospital. The situation was so bad that something had to be done, and with many misgivings, the medical audit method was chosen. The audit showed that the suspicions were ungrounded. A Tissue Committee was set up and the cases in which the pathology report failed to confirm the pre-operative diagnosis were not excessive—they were below the common average of 10%. There were disclosed other deficiencies, of course, which they set about to remedy. The main result was an improvement in staff and community relations because conditions were not nearly so bad as they had seemed, and many dark suspicions were removed. It is the fear of finding out something bad that deters many hospitals from undertaking thorough medical audits—but finding the truth is less painful than the feeling that there are hidden evils. The systematic medical audit brings facts out into the open— and the effect is salutary for all concerned —the patient, the physician, the hospital and the community.

C

J oint Commission's Current List of Indicators for Beta Testing (1992)

Anesthesia Care Indicators for Beta Testing*

AN-1 Indicator (Numerator): Patients developing a CNS complication during or within two postprocedure days of procedures involving anesthesia administration, subcategorized by ASA-PS class, patient age, and CNS vs non-CNS related procedures.

AN-2 Indicator (Numerator): Patients developing a peripheral neurologic deficit during or within two postprocedure days of procedures involving anesthesia administration.

AN-3 Indicator (Numerator): Patients developing an acute myocardial infarction during or within two postprocedure days of procedures involving anesthesia administration, subcategorized by ASA-PS class, patient age, and cardiac vs noncardiac procedures.

AN-4 Indicator (Numerator): Patients with a cardiac arrest during or within one postprocedure day of procedures involving anesthesia administration, excluding patients with required intraoperative cardiac arrest, subcategorized by ASA-PS class, patient age, and cardiac vs noncardiac procedures.

---

*Note: These indicators are subject to revision based on the results of further testing. The Joint Commission recommends that these indicators be considered for use by accredited organizations, but at this time does not require their use.

AN-5 Indicator (Numerator): Patients with unplanned respiratory arrest during or within one postprocedure day involving anesthesia administration.

AN-6 Indicator (Numerator): Death of patients during or within two postprocedure days of procedures involving anesthesia administration, subcategorized by class and patient age.

AN-7 Indicator (Numerator): Unplanned admission of patients to the hospital within one postprocedure day following outpatient procedures involving anesthesia administration.

AN-8 Indicator (Numerator): Unplanned admission of patients to an intensive care unit within one postprocedure day of procedures involving anesthesia administration and with ICU stay greater than one day.

Obstetrical Care Indicators for Beta Testing*

OB-1 Indicator (Numerator): Patients with primary cesarean section for failure to progress.

OB-2 Indicator (Numerator): Patients with attempted vaginal birth after cesarean section (VBAC), subcategorized by success or failure.

OB-3 Indicator (Numerator): Patients with excessive maternal blood loss defined by intrapartum and/or postpartum red blood cell transfusion or a low post-delivery hematocrit or hemoglobin (Hct <22%, Hgb <7 gms) or a significant pre- to post-delivery decrease in hematocrit (>11%) or hemoglobin (>3.5 gms) excluding patients with abruptio placenta or placenta previa.

OB-4 Indicator (Numerator): Patients with the diagnosis of eclampsia.

OB-5 Indicator (Numerator): The delivery of infants weighing less than 2,500 grams following either induction of labor or repeat cesarean section without medical indications.

---

*Note: These indicators are subject to revision based on the results of further testing. The Joint Commission recommends that these indicators be considered for use by accredited organizations, but at this time does not require their use.

OB-6 Indicator (Numerator): Term infants admitted to an NICU within one day of delivery and with NICU stay greater than one day excluding admission for major congenital anomalies.

OB-7 Indicator (Numerator): Neonates with an Apgar score of 3 or less at 5 minutes and a birthweight greater than 1,500 grams.

OB-8 Indicator (Numerator): Neonates with a discharge diagnosis of significant birth trauma.

OB-9 Indicator (Numerator): Term infants with a diagnosis of hypoxic encephalopathy or clinically apparent seizure prior to discharge from the hospital of birth excluding newborns with a diagnosis of fetal alcohol syndrome, and other drug reactions and withdrawal syndromes.

OB-10 Indicator (Numerator): Deaths of infants weighing 500 grams or more subcategorized by intrahospital neonatal deaths, total stillborns, and intrapartum stillborns.

Oncology Indicators for Beta Testing*

Oncology Indicator Patient Population: Inpatients admitted for initial diagnosis and/or treatment of primary lung, colon, rectal, or female breast cancer.

ON-1 Indicator Focus: Availability of data for diagnosis and staging. Indicator (Numerator): Surgical pathology consultation reports (pathology reports) containing histological type, tumor size, status of margins, appropriate lymph node examination, assessment of invasion or extension as indicated, and AJCC/pTN classification for patients with resection for primary cancer of the lung, colon/rectum, or female breast.

ON-2 Indicator Focus: Use of staging by managing physicians. Indicator (Numerator): Patients undergoing treatment for primary cancer of the lung, colon/rectum, or female breast with AJCC stage of tumor designated by a managing physician.

---

*Note: These indicators are subject to revision based on the results of further testing. The Joint Commission recommends that these indicators be considered for use by accredited organizations, but at this time does not require their use.

ON-3 Indicator Focus: Effectiveness of cancer treatment. Indicator (Numerator): Survival of patients with primary cancer of the lung, colon/rectum, or female breast by stage and histologic type.*

ON-4 Indicator Focus: Use of tests critical to diagnosis, prognosis, and clinical management. Indicator (Numerator): Female patients with invasive primary breast cancer undergoing initial biopsy or resection of a tumor larger than one centimeter in greatest dimension who have presence of estrogen receptor diagnostic analysis results in medical record.

ON-5 Indicator Focus: Use of multimodal therapy in treatment and follow-up.* Indicator (Numerator): Female patients with AJCC Stage II pathologic lymph node positive primary invasive breast cancer treated with systemic adjuvant therapy.

ON-6 Indicator Focus: Effectiveness of preoperative diagnosis and staging. Indicator (Numerator): Patients with non–small cell primary lung cancer undergoing thoracotomy with complete surgical resection of tumor.

ON-7 Indicator Focus: Specific clinical events as a means of assessing multiple aspects of surgical care for lung cancers. Indicator (Numerator): Patients undergoing pulmonary resection for primary lung cancer with postoperative complication of empyema, bronchopleural fistula, reoperation for postoperative bleeding, mechanical ventilation greater than 5 days postop, or intrahospital death.

ON-8 Indicator Focus: Comprehensiveness of diagnostic workup. Indicator (Numerator): Patients with resections of primary colorectal cancer whose preoperative evaluation by a managing physician includes examination of the entire colon, liver function tests, chest x-ray, and carcinoembryonic antigen (CEA) levels.

ON-9 Indicator Focus: Documentation of staging, prognosis, and surgical treatment. Indicator (Numerator): Patients with resec-

---

*Efficient mechanisms to obtain postdischarge data will be explored only with a subset of beta test hospitals. Ability to obtain this data during beta testing is not a requirement for participation.

tion of primary colorectal cancer whose operative reports include location of primary tumor, local extent of disease, extent of resection, and assessment of residual abdominal disease.

ON-10 **Indicator Focus:** Use of treatment approaches that impact on quality of life. **Indicator (Numerator):** Patients with primary rectal cancer undergoing abdominoperineal resections with 6 cm or more of free distal surgical margin present on specimen, as documented in surgical pathology gross description.

ON-11 **Indicator Focus:** Interdisciplinary treatment and follow-up. **Indicator (Numerator):** Patients with AJCC Stage II or III primary rectal cancer with documentation of referral to or treatment by a radiation or medical oncologist.

Cardiovascular Indicators for Beta Testing*

Cardiovascular Indicator Patient Population: The cardiovascular indicators draw from four populations described below: coronary artery bypass grafts (CABG), percutaneous transluminal coronary angioplasty (PTCA), acute myocardial infarction (MI), and congestive heart failure (CHF).

CABG Patient Population: Patients undergoing coronary artery bypass grafts (CABG) excluding those with other cardiac or peripheral vascular surgical procedures performed at the time of the CABG (eg, valve replacement).

CV-1 **Indicator Focus:** Intrahospital mortality as a means of assessing multiple aspects of CABG care. **Indicator (Numerator):** Intrahospital mortality of patients undergoing isolated coronary artery bypass graft (CABG) procedures, subcategorized by initial or subsequent CABG procedures, by emergent or non-emergent clinical status, and by postoperative day and intrahospital location of death.

CV-2 **Indicator Focus:** Extended postoperative stay as a means of

---

*Note: These indicators are subject to revision based on the results of further testing. The Joint Commission recommends that these indicators be considered for use by accredited organizations, but at this time does not require their use.

assessing multiple aspects of CABG care. **Indicator (Numerator):** Patients with prolonged postoperative stay for isolated coronary artery bypass graft (CABG) procedures, subcategorized by initial or subsequent CABG procedures, by emergent or non-emergent procedures, and by the use or non-use of a circulatory support device.

PTCA Patient Population: Patients for whom a percutaneous transluminal coronary angioplasty (PTCA) procedure is initiated, regardless of whether or not a lesion is crossed or dilated.

CV-3 **Indicator Focus:** Intrahospital mortality as a means of assessing multiple aspects of PTCA care. **Indicator (Numerator):** Intrahospital mortality of patients following percutaneous transluminal coronary angioplasty (PTCA), subcategorized by emergent or nonemergent clinical status and by postprocedure day and intrahospital location of death.

CV-4 **Indicator Focus:** Specific clinical events as a means of assessing multiple aspects of PTCA care. **Indicator (Numerator):** Patients undergoing nonemergent percutaneous transluminal coronary angioplasty (PTCA) with subsequent occurrence of either an acute myocardial infarction (MI) or coronary artery bypass graft (CABG) procedure within the same hospitalization.

CV-5 **Indicator Focus:** Effectiveness of PTCA. **Indicator (Numerator):** Patients undergoing attempted or completed percutaneous transluminal coronary angioplasty (PTCA) during which any lesion attempted is not dilated.

MI Patient Population: Patients with a principal diagnosis of acute myocardial infarction (MI) either upon hospital discharge, emergency department (ED) transfer to another acute care facility, or death in the emergency department (ED), and patients who are admitted for an acute MI or to rule out an acute MI.

CV-6 **Indicator Focus:** Intrahospital mortality as a means of assessing multiple aspects of acute MI care. **Indicator (Numerator):** Intrahospital mortality of patients with principal discharge diagnosis of acute myocardial infarction (MI), subcategorized by history of previous infarction, age, and intrahospital location of death.

CV-7 Indicator Focus: Diagnostic accuracy and resource utilization. Indicator (Numerator): Patients admitted for acute myocardial infarction (MI), rule-out acute MI, or unstable angina who have a discharge diagnosis of acute MI, subcategorized by admission to an intensive care unit, a monitored bed, or an unmonitored bed.

CHF Patient Population: Patients with a principal discharge diagnosis of congestive heart failure, with or without specific etiologies.

CV-8 Indicator Focus: Diagnostic accuracy. Indicator (Numerator): Patients with principal discharge diagnosis of congestive heart failure (CHF) with documented etiology and chest X-ray substantiation of CHF.

CV-9 Indicator Focus: Monitoring patient's response to therapy. Indicator (Numerator): Patients with a principal discharge diagnosis of congestive heart failure (CHF) and with at least two determinations of patient weight and of serum sodium, potassium, blood urea nitrogen (BUN), and creatinine levels.

Trauma Indicators for Beta Testing*

Trauma Indicator Patient Population: Patients with ICD-9-CM diagnostic code of 800 through 959.9 who are either admitted to the hospital, die in the emergency department (ED), or are transferred from the hospital or the ED to another acute care facility, excluding patients with the following isolated injuries: burns; hip fractures in the elderly; specified fractures of the face, hand, and foot; and specified eye wounds.

TR-1 Indicator Focus: Efficiency of emergency medical services (EMS). Indicator (Numerator): Trauma patients with prehospital emergency medical services (EMS) scene time greater than 20 minutes.

TR-2 Indicator Focus: Ongoing monitoring of trauma patients. Indicator (Numerator): Trauma patients with blood pressure,

---

*Note: These indicators are subject to revision based on the results of further testing. The Joint Commission recommends that these indicators be considered for use by accredited organizations, but at this time does not require their use.

pulse, respiration, and Glasgow Coma Score (GCS) documented in the emergency department (ED) record on arrival and hourly until inpatient admission to operating room or intensive care unit, death, or transfer to another care facility (hourly GCS needed only if altered state of consciousness).

TR-3 **Indicator Focus:** Airway management of comatose trauma patients. **Indicator (Numerator):** Comatose patients discharged from the emergency department (ED) prior to the establishment of a mechanical airway.

TR-4 **Indicator Focus:** Timeliness of diagnostic testing. **Indicator (Numerator):** Trauma patients with diagnosis of intracranial injury and altered state of consciousness upon emergency department (ED) arrival receiving initial head computerized tomography (CT) scan greater than 2 hours after ED arrival.

TR-5 **Indicator Focus:** Timeliness of surgical intervention for adult head injury. **Indicator (Numerator):** Trauma patients with diagnosis of extradural or subdural brain hemorrhage undergoing craniotomy greater than 4 hours after emergency department (ED) arrival (excluding intracranial pressure monitoring), subcategorized by pediatric or adult patients.

TR-6 **Indicator Focus:** Timeliness of surgical intervention for orthopedic injuries. **Indicator (Numerator):** Trauma patients with open fractures of the long bones as a result of blunt trauma receiving initial surgical treatment greater than 8 hours after emergency department (ED) arrival.

TR-7 **Indicator Focus:** Timeliness of surgical intervention for abdominal injuries. **Indicator (Numerator):** Trauma patients with diagnosis of laceration of the liver or spleen, requiring surgery undergoing laparotomy greater than 2 hours after emergency department (ED) arrival, subcategorized by pediatric or adult patients.

TR-8 **Indicator Focus:** Surgical decision making for abdominal gunshot and/or stab wounds. **Indicator (Numerator):** Trauma patients undergoing laparotomy for wounds penetrating the abdominal wall, subcategorized by gunshot and/or stab wounds.

TR-9 Indicator Focus: Timeliness of patient transfers. **Indicator (Numerator):** Trauma patients transferred from initial receiving hospital to another acute care facility within 6 hours from emergency department (ED) arrival to ED departure.

TR-10 Indicator Focus: Surgical decision making for orthopedic injuries. **Indicator (Numerator):** Adult trauma patients with femoral diaphyseal fractures treated by a nonfixation technique.

TR-11 Indicator Focus: Clinical decision making for potentially preventable deaths. **Indicator (Numerator):** Intrahospital mortality of trauma patients with one or more of the following conditions who did not undergo a procedure for the condition: tension pneumothorax, hemoperitoneum, hemothoraces, ruptured aorta, pericardial tamponade, and epidural or subdural hemorrhage.

TR-12 Indicator Focus: Systems necessary for obtaining autopsies for trauma victims. **Indicator (Numerator):** Trauma patients who expired within 48 hours of emergency department (ED) arrival for whom an autopsy was performed.

Infection Control Indicators for Beta Testing*

IC-1 Indicator Focus: Surgical wound infection. **Indicator (Numerator):** Selected inpatient and outpatient surgical procedures complicated by a wound infection during hospitalization or postdischarge.

IC-2 Indicator Focus: Postoperative pneumonia. **Indicator (Numerator):** Selected inpatient surgical procedures complicated by the onset of pneumonia during hospitalization but not beyond 10 postoperative days.

IC-3 Indicator Focus: Urinary catheter usage. **Indicator (Numerator):** Selected surgical procedures on inpatients who are catheterized during the perioperative period.

---

*Note: These indicators are subject to revision based on the results of further testing. The Joint Commission recommends that these indicators be considered for use by accredited organizations, but at this time does not require their use.

IC-4 **Indicator Focus:** Ventilator pneumonia. **Indicator (Numerator):** Ventilated patients who develop pneumonia.

IC-5 **Indicator Focus:** Postpartum endometritis. **Indicator (Numerator):** Inpatients who develop endometritis following cesarean section, followed until discharge.

IC-6 **Indicator Focus:** Concurrent surveillance of primary bloodstream infection. **Indicator (Numerator):** Inpatients with a central or umbilical line who develop primary bloodstream infection.

IC-7 **Indicator Focus:** Medical record abstraction of primary bloodstream infection. **Indicator (Numerator):** Inpatients with a central or umbilical line and primary bloodstream infection, analyzed by method of identification.

IC-8 **Indicator Focus:** Employee health program. **Indicator (Numerator):** Hospital staff who have been immunized for measles (rubeola) or are known to be immune

Medication Use Indicators for Beta Testing*

MU-1 **Indicator Focus:** Individualizing dosage. **Indicator (Numerator):** Inpatients over 65 years old in whom creatinine clearance has been estimated.

MU-2 **Indicator Focus:** Individualizing dosage. **Indicator (Numerator):** Inpatients receiving parenteral aminoglycosides who have a measured aminoglycoside serum level.

MU-3 **Indicator Focus:** Reviewing the order. **Indicator (Numerator):** New medication orders prompting consultation by the pharmacist with physician or nurse subcategorized by orders changed.

MU- 4 **Indicator Focus:** Timing of medication administration. **Indicator (Numerator):** Patients receiving intravenous prophylactic antibiotics within 2 hours before the first surgical incision.

---

*Note: These indicators are subject to revision based on the results of further testing. The Joint Commission recommends that these indicators be considered for use by accredited organizations, but at this time does not require their use.

MU-5 **Indicator Focus:** Accuracy of medication dispensing and administration. **Indicator (Numerator):** Number of reported significant medication errors.

MU-6 **Indicator Focus:** Informing the patient about the medication. **Indicator (Numerator):** Inpatients with principal and/or other diagnoses of insulin dependent diabetes mellitus who demonstrate self-blood glucose monitoring and self-administration of insulin before discharge, or are referred for postdischarge follow-up for diabetes management.

MU-7 **Indicator Focus:** Monitoring patient response. **Indicator (Numerator):** Inpatients receiving digoxin, theophylline, phenytoin, or lithium who have no corresponding measured drug levels or whose highest measured level exceeds a specific limit.

MU-8 **Indicator Focus:** Monitoring patient response. **Indicator (Numerator):** Inpatients receiving warfarin or intravenous therapeutic heparin who also receive vitamin K, protamine sulfate, or fresh frozen plasma.

MU-9 **Indicator Focus:** Reporting adverse drug reactions. **Indicator (Numerator):** ADRs reported through the hospital's ADR reporting system analyzed by method of reporting (spontaneous or retrospective medical record abstraction), type of ADR (dose related or nondose related), and time of occurrence (before admission or during hospitalization).

MU-10 **Indicator Focus:** Reviewing complete drug regimen. **Indicator (Numerator):** Inpatients receiving more than one type of oral benzodiazepine simultaneously.

MU-11 **Indicator Focus:** Reviewing complete drug regimen. **Indicator (Numerator):** Inpatients with seven or more prescribed medications on discharge.

MU-12 **Indicator Focus:** Overall performance of medication use system. **Indicator (Numerator):** Patients less than 25 years old with a principal discharge diagnosis of bronchoconstrictive pulmonary disease, who are readmitted to the hospital or visit the emergency department within 15 days of discharge due to an exacerbation of their principal diagnosis.

Home Infusion Therapy Indicators for Beta Testing*

The Home Infusion Therapy Indicator Development Task Force initially drafted and reviewed 27 indicators. Following discussion about the availability of data in the home care field, and the diverse organizational structures of and services provided by home infusion companies, the Task Force selected the following indicators as a first step toward establishing a national performance database focused on home infusion therapy. Although indicators 1, 2, 3, and 4 all appear to be single indicators, the expectation for data collection encompasses using each of these four indicators for *each* type of infusion therapy provided by the company. Thus, if TPN and antibiotic therapy are provided, there will be *two rates* for each of those four indicators. Subcategory rates defined in these four indicators will also be determined for *each* type of therapy provided. Indicators 5 and 6 are not designed in this manner; there are various subcategories associated with each of them, but they are not initially defined by type of therapy.

Consequently, what appears to be a list of six indicators for home infusion therapy actually translates to a larger number that are applicable to all home infusion providers, regardless of their patient population or therapy mix.

IT-1 **Indicator Focus:** Unscheduled inpatient admission by type of therapy. **Indicator (Numerator):** Clients receiving home infusion therapy who have an unscheduled inpatient admission subcategorized by reason for admission.

IT-2 **Indicator Focus:** Discontinued infusion therapy by type of therapy. **Indicator (Numerator):** Courses of infusion therapy discontinued before prescribed completion, subcategorized by reason for discontinuation.

---

*Note: These indicators are subject to revision based on the results of further testing. The Joint Commission recommends that these indicators be considered for use by accredited organizations, but at this time does not require their use.

IT-3 **Indicator Focus:** Interruption in infusion therapy by type of therapy. **Indicator (Numerator):** Total number of interruptions in infusion therapy subcategorized by reason for interruption in therapy.

IT-4 **Indicator Focus:** Prevention and surveillance of infection by type of therapy. **Indicator (Numerator):** Clients with central lines whose catheter is removed or who receive antibiotic therapy for a confirmed or suspected catheter-related infection subcategorized by type of central line catheter and number of lumens.

IT-5 **Indicator Focus:** Reporting adverse drug reactions. **Indicator (Numerator):** Total number of suspected or confirmed adverse drug reactions (ADRs) experienced by infusion therapy clients, subcategorized by the type and severity of ADR and by drug class.

IT-6 **Indicator Focus:** Client monitoring and appropriate intervention. **Indicator (Numerator):** Clients receiving total parenteral nutrition (TPN) and/or enteral therapy who are achieving or maintaining desired weight.

D

Overview of the Joint Commission's Indicator Development Form (1992)

The Indicator Development Form (IDF) is used to describe and record the developmental process for each indicator. The IDF also provides the necessary information on how to collect and analyze each indicator. A brief statement of the indicator focus precedes the seven sections of the IDF. The Indicator Focus identifies the specific component or aspect of care that the indicator is monitoring. The seven sections of the IDF are listed and described below:

- Section I—Indicator Statement
- Section II—Definition of Terms
- Section III—Type of Indicator
- Section IV—Rationale
- Section V—Description of Indicator Population
- Section VI—Indicator Logic
- Section VII—Underlying Factors

Section I, **Indicator Statement**, describes the function, activity, event or outcome being evaluated. Indicator statements may be simple or complex when qualifiers such as categories or subgroups are introduced.

Section II, **Definition of Terms**, contains selected terms from the indicator statement that may require further explanation to ensure uniform data collection and appropriate analysis. Terms are defined as precisely as possible, including translation into specific and widely accepted terminology such as ICD-9-CM codes. The collection of comparable data and its meaningful analysis and comparison is extremely difficult, if not impossible, without uniform definitions.

Section III, **Type of Indicator**, defines whether the indicator is a sentinel event or rate-based indicator. A sentinel event indicator measures a serious, undesirable, and often avoidable process or outcome that occurs rarely or at a low frequency. Sentinel events are of sufficient gravity to warrant investigation of every occurrence.

A rate-based indicator aggregates events that are expected to occur at some reasonable frequency. Rate-based indicators may measure adverse events or desirable events. The indicator rate of a negative event should ideally move toward 0% over time, whereas a positive event indicator rate should move toward 100%. Further assessment is required if the rate of events shows a significant trend within an institution over time, exceeds a predetermined threshold, or evidences a significant difference when compared to that of peer institutions.

This section also describes whether the indicator measures an outcome or process of patient care. An outcome indicator measures the patient's condition or response with respect to patient care activities or procedures performed or not performed. A process indicator assesses an important and discrete activity that is carried out either to directly care for the patient or to support patient care.

Section IV, **Rationale**, explains why an indicator is thought to be useful in assessing the process or outcome of care measured by the indicator and identifies the components of patient care assessed by the indicator, as determined by task force members. This section also includes selected references that support the rationale.

Section V, **Description of Indicator Population**, identifies the numerator and denominator used to derive the indicator rate. The denominator describes the criteria used to establish the population evaluated by the indicator. The numerator is the portion of the denominator that satisfies the conditions required for indicator membership as described by the indicator statement. The numerator and denominator populations may be further subcategorized by specific attributes of the indicator. The purpose of subcategorizing is to identify more homogeneous populations, allowing for meaningful comparison and analysis of indicator rates across hospitals.

Section VI, **Indicator Logic**, illustrates the steps required to arrive at the indicator numerator and denominator. The indicator logic is displayed in a flowchart format using standard flowchart symbols to depict the processes and decisions required to define the indicator event.

The indicator logic assigns a category to each case evaluated by the indicator. There are five categories describing the relationship of a case to an indicator:

• Category 1 = Eligibility undetermined: Key data elements that determine if the case meets criteria for consideration are missing from the database.

• Category 2 = Ineligible: Sufficient data elements are in the database to determine that the case does not meet the criteria for the specified indicator.

• Category 3 = Potential numerator eligibility: Sufficient data elements are present to determine that the case is at least in the denominator, but there is insufficient data to determine if the case is an indicator event.

• Category 4 = Eligible denominator: Sufficient data are present to determine that the case is in the denominator, but the case is not an indicator case.

• Category 5 = Indicator identified case: Sufficient data are present to determine that the case meets the criteria for an indicator event.

Section VII, **Underlying Factors**, suggests potential causes or contributing factors that may explain variance in indicator data. In order to improve performance, hospitals must first be able to identify the patient, practitioner, organizational, and environmental variables that influence hospital performance and affect patient outcomes. This section is designed to help hospitals begin to understand and interpret their indicator data.

E

Example of Completed Indicator Development Form for Joint Commission Trauma Care Indicator #TR-1: Efficiency of Emergency Medical Services

Trauma Indicator Development Form

TR-1 Indicator Focus: Efficiency of Emergency Medical Services (EMS)

I. Indicator (Numerator)
    Trauma patients with prehospital emergency medical services (EMS) scene times greater than 20 minutes.

II. Definition of Terms
    (Terms contained in the indicator which may be ambiguous or need further explanation for collection purposes.)
    Prehospital (EMS) Scene Time: Interval between arrival of initial emergency personnel (eg, fire department, ambulance, paramedics) and patient departure from the scene of injury to the hospital.

III. Type of Indicator
    A. This is a:
    / / sentinel event indicator (all occurrences warrant investigation;)
    or
    /✔/ rate-based indicator (further assessment warranted if the occurrence rate shows a significant trend, exceeds predetermined thresholds, or indicates significant differences when compared to peer institutions.)

B. This indicator primarily addresses:
/✔/ a process of patient care;
or
/ / a patient outcome.

IV. Rationale

A. Intent of monitoring the indicator event.

The process of patient transportation may be related to outcomes of morbidity and mortality because the condition of critically injured patients frequently deteriorates over time. Thus, except for problems in patient extrication, trauma patients should be transported with minimal delay. Scene times greater than 20 minutes may indicate problems in the quality and/or appropriateness of care provided by prehospital personnel who are not limiting intervention to immediate life-sustaining techniques. High rates of indicator activity in comparison to peer institutions would signal the need for in-depth evaluation.

B. Selected references:

American College of Surgeons, Committee on Trauma: Hospital and prehospital resources for optimal care of the injured patient. *Bulletin of the ACS* Appendix G: No. 2, 1987.

Gervin AS, Fischer RP: The importance of prompt transport and salvage of patients with penetrating heart wounds. *J Trauma* 22:443–8, 1982.

Pons PT, Honigman B, Moore EE, Rosen P, Antuna B, Dernocoeru J. Prehospital advanced trauma life support for critical penetrating wounds to the thorax and abdomen. *J Trauma* 25:828–32, 1985.

Cwinn AA, Pons PT, Moore EE, Marx JA, Honigman B, Dinerman N. Prehospital advanced life support for critical blunt trauma victims. *Ann Emerg Med* 16:399–403, 1987.

C. The components of patient care assessed by this indicator.

1. EMS personnel capability and judgment related to assessment and treatment.

V. Description of Indicator Population

A. Subcategories (patient subpopulations by which the indicator data will be separated for analysis.)
None

B. Indicator Data Format (the manner in which indicator data will be expressed.)
    1. Rate-based indicator format:
        a. Numerator(s): Number of EMS-transported trauma patients with scene times greater than 20 minutes.
        b. Denominator(s): Number of EMS-transported trauma patients.
    2. Sentinel event indicator format: N/A

VI. Indicator Logic
See the flowchart on the next page (Figure 20).

VII. Underlying Factors
Factors not included in the indicator that may account for significant indicator rates or indicator activity.
    A. Patient-based factors (factors outside the health care organization's control contributing to patient outcomes)
        1. Severity of illness (factors related to the degree or stage of disease prior to treatment)
            a. difficult airway control
            b. multiple fractures
            c. traumatic cardiac arrest
        2. Comorbid conditions (disease factors not intrinsic to the primary disease which may have an impact on patient suitability for, or tolerance of, diagnostic or therapeutic care)
            a. disruptive patient
            b. difficult intravenous access
        3. Other patient factors (nondisease factors that may have an impact on care, eg, age, sex, refusal of consent)
            a. problematic extrication
            b. multiple trauma patients
            c. scene control problems
            d. delayed ambulance arrival
            e. patient communication problems

Figure 20

Indicator Logic
Trauma Patients with Prehospital Emergency Medical Services (EMS) Scene Times Greater Than 20 Minutes

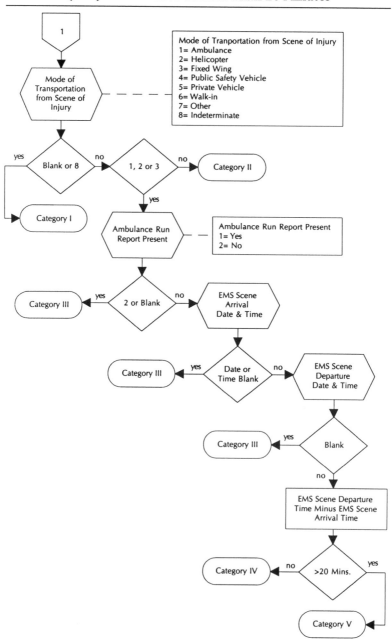

B. Non-patient-based factors

1. Practitioner-based factors (factors related to specific health care practitioners, eg, physicians, nurses, respiratory therapists)

    a. inadequate training or inexperience of prehospital personnel

    b. inappropriate techniques used by prehospital personnel

    c. fatigue or illness of health care practitioners

    d. failure of prehospital personnel to follow protocols

    e. failure to contact or maintain contact with hospital-based medical personnel

2. Organization-based factors (factors related to the health care organization which contribute to either specific aspects of patient care or to the general ability of direct caregivers to provide services)

    a. inadequate or inappropriate standing medical orders

    b. inadequate or inappropriate training of personnel

    c. inadequate ongoing review of personnel performance

    d. equipment malfunction

    e. dispatch to scene of inappropriate or insufficient personnel

    f. inadequate medical control

    g. inadequate supplies

F

Joint Commission's Medication Use and Infection Control Indicator Data Elements Master Lists for Beta Testing Phase

(Data elements 1 through 18 are core data elements and apply to all medication use/infection control indicators.)

1. Medical Record Number
2. Admission Date
3. Time of Admission
4. Admission Source
5. Type of Admission
6. Discharge Date
7. Time of Discharge
8. Discharge Disposition
9. Date of Birth
10. Sex
11. Race and Ethnicity
12. Zip Code
13. Marital Status
14. Expected Principal Source of Payment
15. Principal ICD-9-CM Diagnosis at Discharge
16. Other ICD-9-CM Diagnoses at Discharge
17. Principal ICD-9-CM Procedure and Principal Procedure Date
18. Other ICD-9-CM Procedures and Dates
19. Parenteral Aminoglycoside (MU-1)
20. Serum Drug Level (MU-1)
21. Estimated Creatinine Clearance (MU-2)
22. Serum Creatinine Measured (MU-2)

23. New Medication Orders Received by Pharmacy (MU-3)
24. New Medication Orders Prompting Consultation by Physician or Nurse (MU-3)
25. New Medication Orders Prompting Consultation Resulted in a Change in Order (Orders Changed) (MU-3)
26. Was Select Procedure Performed? (MU-4)
27. Selected Surgical Procedure (MU-4)
28. Prophylactic Antibiotic Administered (MU-4)
29. Antibiotic Administration Date (MU-4)
30. Antibiotic Administration Time (MU-4)
31. Date Surgical Procedure (MU-4)
32. Surgery Start Time (MU-4)
33. Doses Dispensed (MU-5)
34. Medication Errors Totals (MU-5)
    Omission
    Unauthorized Drug
    Wrong Dose
35. Insulin Dependent Diabetes Mellitus (MU-6)
36. Demo Self Blood Glucose Monitoring (MU-6)
37. Demo of Self-administration of Insulin (MU-6)
38. Postdischarge Follow-up Referral (MU-6)
39. Received Digoxin (MU-7)
40. Received Theophylline (MU-7)
41. Received Phenytoin (MU-7)
42. Received Lithium (MU-7)
43. Digoxin Level Measured (MU-7)
44. Theophylline Level Measured (MU-7)
45. Phenytoin Level Measured (MU-7)
46. Lithium Level Measured (MU-7)
47. Highest Digoxin Level Exceeds 3.0 ng/ml (MU-7)
48. Highest Theophylline Level Exceeds 20 mcg/ml (MU-7)
49. Highest Phenytoin Level Exceeds 20 mcg/ml (MU-7)
50. Highest Lithium Level Exceeds 1.4 mC (MU-7)
51. Receiving Anticoagulant: Intravenous Therapeutic Heparin, Warfarin (MU-8)
52. Start Date of Anticoagulant (MU-8)
53. Receiving Antidote: Vitamin K, Protamine Sulfate, Fresh Frozen Plasma (MU-8)

54. Start Date of Antidote (MU-8)
55. ADRs Reported (MU-9)
56. Dose-Related ADRs (MU-9)
57. Non-dose Related ADRs (MU-9)
58. ADRs Occurring Prior to Admission (MU-9)
59. ADRs Occurring During Hospitalization (MU-9)
60. ADRs Reported Through the Spontaneous Reporting System (MU-9)
61. ADRs Reported Retrospectively (MU-9)
62. ADRs Reported Both Spontaneously and Retrospectively (MU-9)
63. Total Hospital Discharges (MU-9, MU-1)
64. Patient Has Active Order for Benzodiazepine (MU-10)
65. Receiving at Least One Oral Benzodiazepine (MU-10)
66. Name of Oral Benzodiazepine Received (See Definition of Terms for a comprehensive list) (MU-10)
67. Start Date of Each Oral Benzodiazepine (MU-10)
68. Stop Date of Each Oral Benzodiazepine (MU-10)
69. Number of Medications Prescribed at Discharge (MU-11)
70. Type of Return Visit (MU-12)
71. Reason for Return Visit Related to Respiratory Condition (MU-12)
72. Date of Return Visit (MU-12)
73. Discharge Date of Last Hospitalization (MU-12)

Infection Control Indicator Data Elements

(Data elements 1 through 18 are core data elements and apply to all medication use/infection control indicators.)

1. Medical Record Number
2. Admission Date
3. Time of Admission
4. Admission Source
5. Type of Admission
6. Discharge Date
7. Time of Discharge
8. Discharge Disposition
9. Date of Birth
10. Sex
11. Race and Ethnicity
12. Zip Code

13. Marital Status
14. Expected Principal Source of Payment
15. Principal ICD-9-CM Diagnosis at Discharge
16. Other ICD-9-CM Diagnoses at Discharge
17. Principal ICD-9-CM Procedure and Principal Procedure Date
18. Other ICD-9-CM Procedures and Procedure Dates
19. Was Selected Procedure Performed? (IC-1,2,3)
20. Type of Patient (IC-1,2,3)
21. Selected Surgical Procedure (IC-1,2,3)
22. Date of Surgical Procedure (IC-1,2,3)
23. Time of First Surgical Incision (IC-1,2,3)
24. Surgery Stop Time (IC-1,2,3)
25. ASA Class (IC-1,2)
26. Wound Class (IC-1,2)
27. Incision into the Abdominal Cavity (IC-1)
28. Use of Prophylactic Antibiotic (IC-1,5)
29. Date of Prophylactic Antibiotic Use (IC-1,5)
30. Time of Prophylactic Antibiotic Use (IC-1,5)
31. Number of Admission Diagnoses (IC-1)
32. Evidence of Surgical Wound Infection During Hospitalization (IC-1)
33. Date Surgical Wound Infection Identified (IC-1)
34. Postdischarge Surveillance Initiated (IC-1)
35. Patient Respond to Postdischarge Survey (IC-1)
36. Evidence of Surgical Wound Infection Through Postdischarge Surveillance (IC-1)
37. Incision into Chest, Brain, Mediastinum or Peritoneal Cavity (IC-2)
38. Preoperative Presence of COPD (IC-2)
39. Postoperative Ventilator Support (IC-2)
40. Signs or Symptoms of Pneumonia (IC-2,4)
41. Date of Pneumonia Onset (IC-2,4)
42. Urinary Catheter Inserted (IC-3)
43. Catheter Type Used (IC-3)
44. Date of Catheter Insertion (IC-3)
45. Date of Catheter Removal (IC-4)
46. Was Patient on Ventilator? (IC-4)
47. Date Ventilation Initiated (IC-4)

48. Date Ventilation Discontinued (IC-4)
49. Type of Unit (IC-4,6,7)
50. Other Type of ICU (IC-4,6,7)
51. Date of Unit Admission (IC-4,6,7)
52. Did Patient Have Cesarean Section? (IC-5)
53. Date of Cesarean Section (IC-5)
54. Signs or Symptoms or Diagnosis of Endometritis (IC-5)
55. Date of Signs or Symptoms or Diagnosis of Endometritis (IC-5)
56. Date of First Notation in Patient Record (IC-5)
57. Did Patient Have a Central/Umbilical Line Inserted? (IC-6,7)
58. Type of Line Inserted (IC-6,7)
59. Date of Line Insertion (IC-6,7)
60. Date of Line Removal (IC-6,7)
61. Signs or Symptoms or Diagnosis of Primary Bloodstream Infection (IC-6,7)
62. Date of Signs or Symptoms or Diagnosis of Primary Bloodstream Infection (IC-6,7)
63. Primary Bloodstream Infection Identified During Concurrent Surveillance (IC-7)
64. Primary Bloodstream Infection Identified Through Medical Record Abstraction (IC-IC-7)
65. Total Hospital Staff (IC-8)
66. Total Hospital Staff Immunized or Known to Be Immune to Measles (IC-8)

G

Joint Commission Indicator Development Task Force Members

Anesthesia Care Indicator Development Task Force

Ronald Gabel, MD (Chairperson)
Professor and Chairman
University of Rochester Medical Center
Rochester, NY

Jeffrey Beutler, CRNA, MS
Deputy Executive Director
Anesthesia Profressional Associates
Grand Rapids, MI

Paul DeBruine, MD
Chief of Anesthesiology
Decatur Memorial Hospital
Decatur, IL

Burton S. Epstein, MD
Professor of Anesthesiology
George Washington University Medical Center
Washington, DC

Alvin Hackel, MD
Professor of Anesthesia and Pediatrics
Stanford Medical Center
Stanford, CA

M.T. Jenkins, MD
Chairman Emeritus & Professor of Anesthesiology
Southwestern Medical Center at Dallas
Dallas, TX

Fredrick K. Orkin, MD
Chief of Anesthesia Service
Veterans Affairs Medical Center
White River Junction, VT

Ellison C. Pierce, Jr, MD
Chairman, Department of Anesthesiology
New England Deaconess Hospital
Boston, MA

William R. Wallace, DDS, MSC
University Hospital
Columbus, OH

Christine Zambricki, CRNA, MS
Director of Nurse Anesthesia/PACU
William Beaumont Hospital
Royal Oaks, MI

Cardiovascular Care Indicator Development Task Force

Thomas D. Giles, MD (Chairman)
Director
Cardiovascular Research Laboratory
Louisiana State University Medical Center
New Orleans, LA

John Albers, MD, FACS
Associate Clinical Professor
University of Cincinnati Medical Center
Cincinnati, OH

Elliot L. Cohen, MD
Chief, Emergency and Ambulatory Services
Beverly Hospital
Beverly, MA

Marvin I. Dunn, MD
Director
Division of Cardiovascular Diseases
University of Kansas Medical Center
Kansas City, KS

William Gay, Jr, MD
Professor & Chairman
Department of Surgery
University of Utah School of Medicine
Salt Lake City, UT

Rolf M. Gunnar, MD, FACP, FRCP (Edin)
Gunnar Medical Group
Riverside, IL

Robert H. Jones, MD
Mary and Deryl Hart Professor of Surgery
Duke University Medical Center
Durham, NC

Barry T. Katzen, MD, FACR, FACC
Medical Director
Miami Vascular Institute
Baptist Hospital of Miami
Miami, FL

Spencer B. King, III, MD
Director
Interventional Cardiology
Emory University Hospital
Atlanta, GA

Suzanne B. Knoebel, MD
Professor of Medicine
Indiana University School of Medicine
Krannert Institute of Cardiology
Indianapolis, IN

Ann Schmitt
Consultant
Quality Assurance and Utilization Management
Sugar Land, TX

Joseph Skom, MD, FACP
Chicago, IL

William B. Stason, MD, MSci
Vice President
Health Economics Research
Waltham, MA

Suzanne K. White, RN, MN, CCRN
Director
Department of Cardiovascular Nursing
Emory Hospital
Atlanta, GA

Michael Lesch, MD (Consultant)
Chairman
Department of Medicine
Henry Ford Hospital
Detroit, MI

Gotlieb C. Frieseinger, II, MD (Former Member)
Director
Division of Cardiology
Vanderbilt University School of Medicine
Nashville, TN

Floyd D. Loop, MD (Former Member)
Chairman
Department of Thoracic & Cardiovascular Surgery
Cleveland, OH

John Waldhausen, MD (Former Member)
Chairman
Department of Surgery
Pennsylvania State University
Hershey, PA

Depressive Disorders Indicator Development Task Force

Roger G. Kathol, MD (Chairman)
Associate Professor
Psychiatry and Internal Medicine
University of Iowa
Iowa City, IA

Ivo Abraham, PhD, RN, FAAN
Director
Center on Aging and Health
University of Virginia
Charlottesville, VA

Bonnie Jeanne Benzies, PhD
Administrative Psychologist
Department of Mental Health and Developmental Disabilities
State of Illinois
Hanover Park, IL

Paula J. Clayton, MD
Professor and Head
Department of Psychiatry
University of Minnesota Medical School
Minneapolis, MN

Dian Carswell Cox
Program Services Specialist
Advocacy, Incorporated
Austin, TX

Elizabeth Baker Devereaux, MSW, ACSW/L, OTR/L, FAOTA
Associate Professor
Department of Psychiatry
Marshall University School of Medicine
Huntington, WV

Michael A. Fauman, PhD, MD
Associate Professor
Department of Psychiatry
University of Maryland

Gladys Walton Hall, PhD
Associate Professor
Howard University School of Social Work
Washington, DC

Eva Hernandez, RN, MSN
Community Services Director
Mental Health Coordinator
Erie Family Health Center
Centro de Salud Erie
Chicago, IL

Robert M.A. Hirschfeld, MD
Professor and Chairman
Department of Psychiatry and Behavioral Sciences
University of Texas Medical Branch
Galveston, TX

John S. Lyons, PhD
Associate Professor of Psychiatry, Medicine, and Psychology
Northwestern University Medical School
Chicago, IL

Gary Phillips, STD
Central Regional Director, AAP Mental Health Resources
Instructor in Psychology
Northwestern University
Evanston, IL

Donald M. Steinwachs, PhD
Director
Center on Organization and Financing of
   Care to the Severely Mentally Ill
The Johns Hopkins University
Baltimore, MD

Thomas R. Zastowny, PhD
Director of Quality Assurance and Training
Park Ridge Mental Health Center
Rochester, NY

John S. Zil, MD, MPH, JD
President
American Association of Mental Health Professionals in Corrections
Sacramento, CA

Home Infusion Therapy Indicator Development Task Force

Ruth A. Fisk, RN, MS (Chairperson)
Vice President of Professional Practice
Chartwell Home Therapies
Waltham, MA

Marvin E. Ament, MD
Professor of Pediatrics
UCLA Medical Center
Los Angeles, CA

Jacqueline Birmingham, RN, MS
Director of Discharge Planning
Hartford Hospital
Hartford, CT

Laylee M. Charlang, RN, BSN, OCN
Quality Assurance Coordinator
OPTION Care, Inc
Chico, CA

Kathleen S. Crocker, MSN, RN, CNA, CNSN
National Director of Nursing Services
Critical Care America
Westborough, MA

Wanda Hain Howell, PhD, RD
Assistant Professor
Department of Nutrition and Food Science
University of Arizona
Phoenix, AZ

Jane W. Kwan
Coordinator
Pharmacy Alternate Delivery Programs
The University of Texas
Houston, TX

Karen Martin, RN, MSN, FAAN
Director of Research
The Visiting Nurse Association
Omaha, NE

Sue Masoorli, RN
President, CEO
Perivascular Nurse Consultants
Rockridge, PA

Roberta Rae McAbee, RN, MSN
Registered Nurse
Seattle, WA

Barbara A. McCann
Director
Quality Assurance
Caremark, Inc
Lincolnshire, IL

Jay M. Mirtallo, MS, RPh
Clinical Pharmacist
Nutrition Support Service
The Ohio State University Hospital
Columbus, OH

Sonja A. Nisson, RPh
Clinical Pharmacist
Home Parenteral Care
Grants Pass, OR

Lawrence A. Robinson, MS, PharmD
Chief Operating Officer
PharmaThera, Inc
Memphis, TN

Ezra Steiger, MD
Department of General Surgery
Cleveland Clinic Foundation
Cleveland, OH

Lydia Tanner, MS, RN
Clinical Nurse Specialist/QA Coordinator
Rush Home Health Service
Chicago, IL

Elizabeth V. Tucker
Effective Living Techniques
Minneapolis, MN

David Neville Williams, MD
Park Nicollet Center
Minneapolis, MN

J. Scott Reid, PharmD (Consultant)
Home Health Care and Pharmacy Services
Glen Ellyn, IL

Infection Control Indicator Development Task Force

Robert W. Haley, MD (Chairman)
Southwestern Medical School
University of Texas Health Service Center
Dallas, TX

Darnell Abbott, RN, MPH, CIC
Infection Control
Past President, APIC
Lubbock, TX

Carol J. Applegeet, MSN
Past President, AORN
Highlands Ranch, CO

Dennis Brimhall, MM
President, University Hospital
University of Colorado
Denver, CO

Robert E. Condon, MD, MS, FACS
Department of Surgery
The Medical College of Wisconsin
Milwaukee, WI

Theodore C. Eickhoff, MD
Director of Internal Medicine
Presbyterian/Saint Luke's
Center for Health Sciences Education
Denver, CO

Walter J. Hierholzer, Jr, MD
Director Hospital Epidemiology Program
Yale-New Haven Hospital
New Haven, CT

Douglas C. Hubner, MD
Medical Director of Clinical Pathology
Hillcrest Medical Center
Tulsa, OK

William Jarvis, MD
Chief, Epidemiology Branch
Centers for Disease Control
Atlanta, GA

Elaine L. Larson, PhD, RN, CIC
Nutting Chair in Clinical Nursing
The Johns Hopkins University
Baltimore, MD

R. Michael Massanari, MD, MS
Hospital Epidemiology
Henry Ford Hospital
Detroit, MI

Linda L. McDonald, MSPH, RN, CIC
Infection Control Practitioner
Veterans Administration Medical Center
Seattle, WA

John A. Molinari, PhD
Professor and Chairman
Department of Microbiology and Biochemistry
University of Detroit
Detroit, MI

Ronald Lee Nichols, MD
Henderson Professor of Surgery
Tulane University School of Medicine
New Orleans, LA

Terri Rearick, RN, CIC
Infection Control Coordinator
St Mary's Medical Center
St Luke's Hospital
Racine, WI

Eva N. Skinner, RN
Member-Board of Directors
American Association of Retired Persons
National Office
Washington, DC

Steven Weinstein, MPH, CIC
Infection Control Department
University of Massachusetts Medical Center
Worcester, MA

Medication Use Indicator Development Task Force

Arthur J. Atkinson, Jr, MD (Chairman)
Director of Clinical Pharmacology
Northwestern Memorial Hospital
Chicago, IL

P. Mardi Atkins, BSN, RN
Quality Assurance Coordinator
The Cleveland Clinic Foundation
Cleveland, OH

Kenneth Barker, PhD
Head of Department of Pharmacy Care Systems
Auburn University
Auburn, AL

George W. Belsey
Executive Vice President
American Hospital Association
Chicago, IL

Cheston M. Berlin, MD
University Professor of Pediatrics
Professor of Pharmacology
Chief, Division of General Pediatrics
The Milton S. Hershey Medical Center
Hershey, PA

Sandra B. Fielo, EdD, RN, C
Associate Professor
State University of New York
Brooklyn, NY

Robert O. Friedel, MD
Chairman
Department of Psychiatry & Behavioral Neurobiology
University of Alabama at Birmingham
Birmingham, AL

Anderson Hedberg, MD
Rush-Presbyterian-St Luke's Hospital
Chicago, IL

Anne B. Jackson, RN
American Association of Retired Persons
Washington, DC

Christa L. Jackson, RRA
Baxter Health Care Corp
Grand Prairie, TX

Judith K. Jones, MD, PhD
President
The Deggie Group, Ltd
Arlington, VA

David Kornhauser, MD
DuPont Pharmaceutical Co
Newark, DE

Henri R. Manasse, Jr, PhD
Dean and Professor
University of Illinois at Chicago
Chicago, IL

Cathy Stratton, RN
St Michael's Hospital
Milwaukee, WI

Brian L. Strom, MD, MPH
Associate Professor of Medicine in Pharmacology
University of Pennsylvania School of Medicine
Philadelphia, PA

Bruce Vinson, Pharm D
Director of Pharmacy
Harper Hospital
Detroit, MI

John A. Yagiela, DDS, PhD
Associate Dean for Academic and Administrative Affairs
UCLA School of Dentistry
Los Angeles, CA

David M. Angaran, MS (Consultant)
Professor and Department Chairman, and
Associate Director of Pharmacy at Shands
University of Florida
Gainesville, FL

Obstetrical Care Indicator Development Task Force

C. Irving Meeker, MD (Chairman)
Associate Chairman of Obstetrics and Gynecology
Maine Medical Center
Portland, ME

Helen Varney Burst, CNM
Professor Midwifery Program
Yale University School of Nursing
New Haven, CT

Eric Knox, MD
Director of Perinatal Center
Abbott Northwestern Hospital
Minneapolis, MN

George A. Little, MD
Chairman, Department of Maternal and Child Health
Dartmouth Hitchcock Medical Center
Lebanon, NH

Hubert A. Ritter, MD, FACS
Clinical Professor of Gynecology and Obstetrics
St Luke's University
St Louis, MO

Richard G. Roberts, MD, JD
Associate Professor
Department of Family Medicine
University of Wisconsin
Madison, WI

Anne Scupholme, BA, CNM
Chief Nurse Midwife
Jackson Memorial Hospital
Womens Hospital Center
Miami, FL

William N. Spellacy, MD
Professor and Chairman
Department of OBGYN
University of South Florida College of Medicine
Tampa, FL

Geoffrey Suszkowski, DPS
Administrator of Thoracic Cardiovascular Surgery
The Cleveland Clinic Center
Cleveland, OH

Bonnie Wiltse, RN, MPH
Maternal/Child Health Administration
St Luke's Regional Medical Center
Sioux City, IA

Oncology Care Indicator Development Task Force

John W. Yarbro, MD, PhD (Chairman)
Medical Director
Memorial Medical Center
Springfield, IL

Paul Carbone, MD
Director
Wisconsin Clinical Cancer Center
Madison, WI

Connie G. Creitz, LPN, CTR
Cancer Program Coordinator
Valley Medical Center
Renton, WA

Robert Enck, MD
Medical Director
Cancer Program
Davenport, IA

L. Penfield Faber, MD
Dean of Surgery
Rush-Presbyterian-St Luke's Medical Center
Chicago, IL

Irvin Fleming, MD
Chief Surgical Services
St Jude's Children's Hospital
Memphis, TN

Leslie Ford, MD
Chief
Community Oncology and Rehabilitation Branch
National Cancer Institute
Bethesda, MD

Margaret Hanson Frogge, RN
Executive Vice President of Administration
Riverside Medical Center
Kankakee, IL

Gerald Hanks, MD, FACR
Chairman, Department of Radiation Therapy
Fox Chase Cancer Center
Philadelphia, PA

Kay Horsch
Chairman of the Board
American Cancer Society
Atlanta, GA

Robert V.P. Hutter, MD
Chairman, Department of Pathology
St Barnabas Medical Center
Livingston, NJ

Lisa Lattal-Ogorzalek, JD, MHA
Ambulatory Services Manager
Johns Hopkins Oncology Center
Baltimore, MD

L. Jeremy Miransky, PhD
Quality Assurance/Patient Services
Hospital Review Systems
Memorial Sloan-Kettering Cancer Center
New York, NY

Marvin M. Romsdahl, MD, PhD
Professor of Surgery
The University of Texas
M.D. Anderson Cancer Center
Houston, TX

Raymond Weiss, MD
Chief, Medical Oncology
Walter Reed Army Medical Center
Washington, DC

David Winchester, MD, FACS
Chief, Surgical Oncology
Evanston Hospital
Evanston, IL

B. Hugh Buff, MD, FACP
Surveyor Observer
San Diego, CA

Sigmund Weitzman, MD (Consultant)
Northwestern Memorial Hospital
Chicago, IL

Dolores K. Michels, CTR (Former Member)
King Faisal Specialist Hospital & Research Centre
Kingdom of Soudi Arabia

Trauma Care Indicator Development Task Force

Frank R. Lewis, Jr, MD (Chairman)
Department of Surgery
Henry Ford Hospital
Detroit, MI

John W. Ashworth, MHA
Senior Vice President, Planning
University of Maryland Medical Systems
Baltimore, MD

Yoran Ben-Menachem, MD
Professor and Vice Chairman
UMDNJ, New Jersey Medical School
Newark, NJ

Ellis S. Caplan, MD
Chief of Infectious Diseases
Maryland Institute for Emergency Medicine Services Systems
University of Maryland-Shock Treatment Unit
Baltimore, MD

Howard R. Champion, MD
Director, Surgical Critical Care & Emergency Services
Washington Hospital Center
Washington, DC

H. Barrie Fairley, MB, BS
Professor and Chairman
Stanford University School of Medicine
Stanford, CA

Thomas A. Gennarelli, MD
Vice Chairman
Department of Neurosurgery
University of Pennsylvania
Philadelphia, PA

Robert Heilig, RN, JD
Consultant
Emergency and Trauma Systems
Sacramento, CA

Lenworth M. Jacobs, Jr, MD, MPH
Professor of Surgery, University of Connecticut
Director, Trauma Program/Emergency Medicine
Hartford Hospital
Hartford, CT

Gene W. Kallsen, MD, MPA
Chief of Emergency Medicine
Valley Medical Center
Fresno, CA

Charles L. Rice, MD
Professor and Chairman, Division of General Surgery
The University of Texas
Southwestern Medical Center at Dallas
Dallas, TX

J. David Richardson, MD
Professor & Vice Chairman
Department of Surgery
University of Louisville
Louisville, KY

Ronald Rosenthal, MD
Chief, Division of Trauma
Long Island Jewish Medical Center
New Hyde Park, NY

Nancy L. Siefert, RN, BS
Administrative Director Emergency Care
St Elizabeth's Medical Center
Youngstown, OH

Mark Smith, MD
Professor & Chairman
Department of Emergency Medicine
George Washington University Medical Center
Washington, DC

Joseph J. Tepas, III, MD
Professor and Chief
Division of Pediatric Surgery
University of Florida Health Science Center
Jacksonville, FL

Charles C. Wolferth, Jr, MD
Surgeon-in-Chief
Department of Surgery
Pepper Pavillion
Philadelphia, PA

Margaret O'Leary, MD (Consultant)
St Charles, IL

Glossary

abruptio placenta   Premature detachment of a placenta, often attended by maternal systemic reactions in the form of shock, oliguria, and fibrinogenopenia.

acute myocardial infarction   Necrosis of tissue in the myocardium that results from insufficient blood supply to the heart.

Agenda for Change   The Joint Commission research and development initiative designed to make continuous improvement in patient outcomes and organizational performance the central and explicit objective of Joint Commission accreditation activities. It was initiated in 1987 and encompasses a recasting of Joint Commission standards to emphasize performance of important functions, improvements in survey and decision-making processes, and creation of a national accreditation reference data system based on well-tested indicators of organization performance.

aggregate data indicator   A performance measure based on collection and aggregation of data about many events or phenomena. The events or phenomena may be desirable or undesirable, and the data may be reported as a continuous variable or a discrete variable. The two major types of aggregate data indicators are discrete variable indicators (also called rate-based indicators) and continuous variable indicators.

AJCC   *See* American Joint Committee on Cancer pathologic stage classification and staging system.

alpha phase of indicator testing process   First phase of the Joint Commission's indicator testing process, consisting of the evaluation of indicators' face validity (that is, the ease with which individual indicators can be understood, their relevance for potential users, and their potential as performance measurement tools) and indicator data issues (that is, the degree of indicator data availability, variations in indicator terms and definitions, sources of indicator data, ability of organizations to collect indicator data, access to and ability to retrieve indicator data, and degree of indicator data accuracy).

American Joint Committee on Cancer (AJCC) pathologic stage classification and staging system   A method of describing the extent of cancer based on the pathologic examination of a resected specimen. The pathologic stages are AJCC stages I through V: pT is the pathologic assessment of the primary tumor; pN is the pathologic assessment of the regional lymph nodes.

American Society of Anesthesiologists-Physical Status (ASA-PS) classification system   A system of classifying patients into categories based on the presence and severity of disease: ASA-P1, a normal healthy patient; P2, a patient with mild systemic disease; P3, a patient with severe systemic disease; P4, a patient with severe systemic disease that is a constant threat to life; P5, a moribund patient who is not expected to survive; P6, a declared brain-dead patient whose organs are being removed for donor purposes. An emergency patient in one of the classes above whose procedure is performed on an emergency basis, is designated with an "E" following classification, for example, P2E.

angioplasty   An angiographic procedure for elimination of areas of narrowing in blood vessels.

anticoagulant therapy   Treatment of patients with substances that prevent blood from clotting, such as warfarin and/or intravenous heparin.

appropriateness   A performance dimension concerning the degree to which the care/intervention provided is relevant to the patient's clinical needs, given the current state of knowledge.

ASA-PS   *See* American Society of Anesthesiologists-Physical Status classification system.

assignable cause variation *See* variation, special cause.

asthma A clinical syndrome characterized by increased responsiveness of the tracheobronchial tree to a variety of stimuli. The primary physiologic manifestation of this hyperresponsiveness is variable airway obstruction. These changes are reversible either spontaneously or as a result of therapy.

attributable cause variation *See* variation, special cause.

availability A performance dimension concerning the degree to which the care/intervention is available to meet the needs of the patient served.

average *See* mean.

benchmark A point of reference or standard by which something can be measured or judged, as in benchmarks of performance.

benchmarking A process of measuring a similar organization's product or service according to specified standards in order to compare it with and improve one's own product or service.

benzodiazepine Any of a group of minor tranquilizers, including diazepam, having a common molecular structure and similar pharmacologic activities, such as antianxiety, muscle relaxing, and sedative and hypnotic effects.

beta phase of indicator testing process Second phase of the Joint Commission's indicator testing process, consisting of the assessment of the capacity of a large number of health care organizations to collect and transmit indicator data to the Joint Commission; the ability of the Joint Commission to receive, analyze, and feed back the data; how information related to indicator data may be incorporated into the accreditation process; the reliability and validity of indicators, and the value of indicators (costs and usefulness).

blunt trauma *See* trauma, blunt.

brainstorming A process used to elicit a large number of ideas from a group of people encouraged to use their collective thinking power to generate ideas and unrestrained thoughts in a relatively short period of time.

CABG procedure   *See* coronary artery bypass graft procedure.

cardiac arrest   Sudden cessation of cardiac function, with disappearance of arterial blood pressure, connoting either ventricular fibrillation or ventricular standstill.

cardiac catheterization   An invasive procedure consisting of the passage of a catheter through a vein into the heart for diagnostic purposes.

cardiopulmonary resuscitation (CPR)   The administration of artificial heart and lung action in the event of cardiac and/or respiratory arrest. The two major components of cardiopulmonary resuscitation are artificial ventilation and closed-chest cardiac massage.

cause-and-effect diagram   A pictorial display drawn to represent the relationship between some effect and all the possible causes influencing it; also called "fishbone diagram" because of its appearance and "Ishikawa diagram" after Kaoru Ishikawa, who first developed and applied the tool.

cesarean section or cesarean delivery   Delivery of the fetus through incisions in the abdominal wall (laparotomy) and the uterine wall (hysterotomy). This definition does not include removal of the fetus from the abdominal cavity in case of rupture of the uterus or abdominal pregnancy.

chance variation   *See* variation, chance.

chemotherapy   The administration of any chemical to treat cancer tissue that is not considered to achieve its effect through a change in the hormonal balance.

CHF   *See* congestive heart failure.

chronic obstructive pulmonary disease (COPD)   A disorder characterized by abnormal tests of expiratory flow that do not change markedly over several months of observation; includes emphysema, peripheral airway disease, and chronic bronchitis.

clinical privileges   Authorization granted by the governing body to a practitioner to provide specific patient care services in the organization within defined limits, based on an individual practitioner's license, education, training, experience, competence, health status, and judgment.

coma   A state of unconsciousness from which an individual cannot be aroused even by powerful stimulation; Glasgow Coma Scale score of 8 or less.

common cause variation   *See* variation, common cause.

comorbidity/comorbidities   Disease(s) or condition(s) present at the same time as the principal disease or condition of a patient. Comorbidities are patient-based sources of performance variation that may have an impact on patient suitability for, or tolerance of, diagnostic and/or therapeutic care.

computerized axial tomography (CAT)   The recording of internal body images at a predetermined plane by means of the emergent x-ray beam that is measured by a scintillation counter; the electronic impulses are recorded on a magnetic disk and then are processed by a minicomputer for reconstruction display of the body in cross-section on a cathode ray tube.

congestive heart failure (CHF)   A clinical syndrome characterized by distinctive symptoms and signs resulting from disturbances in cardiac output or from increased venous pressure. Most often applied to myocardial failure with increased pressures distending the ventrical (high end-diastolic pressure) and a cardiac output inadequate for the body's needs; often subclassified as right- or left-sided heart failure depending on whether the systemic or pulmonary veins are predominantly distended.

consensus   Agreement, especially in opinion.

continuity   A performance dimension concerning the degree to which the care/intervention for the patient is coordinated among practitioners, between organizations, and across time.

continuous variable   A measurement that can fall anywhere along a continuous scale.

continuous variable indicator   An aggregate data indicator in which the value of each measurement can fall anywhere along a continuous scale (for example, the length of sticks in inches).

control chart A graphic representation of an attribute of a process, showing plotted values of some statistic gathered from that attribute, and one or two control limits. It has two basic uses: as a basis for judging whether a process is in control, and as an aid in achieving and maintaining statistical control.

control limit The expected limits (upper and/or lower) of common cause variation statistically calculated based on deviations from the process average. Control limits are not specification or tolerance limits.

COPD *See* chronic obstructive pulmonary disease.

coronary artery bypass graft (CABG) procedure A surgical procedure in which a vein or an artery is used to bypass a constricted portion of one or more coronary arteries.

CPR *See* cardiopulmonary resuscitation.

credentialing The process of determining an individual's license, education, training, experience, competence, health status, and judgment in order to render decisions about appointment/ reappointment to the medical staff and the granting/renewal/ revision of clinical privileges.

credentials Evidence of an individual's license, education, training, experience, competence, health status, and judgment.

data The collection of material or facts on which a discussion or an inference is based, such as data in the patient's medical record or indicator data.

data, measurement *See* measurement data.

data accuracy The degree to which data are free of mistakes.

data analysis The process of interpreting aggregated and displayed data and drawing valid conclusions leading to a determination or judgment.

database An organized, comprehensive collection of data.

data completeness The degree to which desired data exist and are available for use.

data element A single piece of data that can be aggregated in a manner with other data elements to identify occurrences of the indicator event targeted for monitoring.

data pattern An identifiable arrangement of data that suggests a design or orderly formation relative to a data set.

data trend One type of data pattern consisting of the general direction of data measurements.

delineation of clinical privileges The process of listing the specific clinical privileges an organization's staff member may be granted.

diabetes mellitus, insulin-dependent Type I diabetes mellitus, characterized by abrupt onset of symptoms, insulinopenia, dependence on exogenous insulin to sustain life, and a tendency to develop ketoacidosis. The peak age of onset is 12 years, but onset can occur at any age. The disorder is due to lack of insulin production by the beta cells of the pancreatic islets. The beta cell injury is associated with viral infection, autoimmune reactions, and (probably) genetic factors.

diagnosis A scientifically or medically acceptable term given to a complex of symptoms (disturbances of function or sensation of which the patient is aware), signs (disturbances the physician or another individual can detect), and findings (detected by laboratory, x-ray, or other diagnostic procedures, or responses to therapy).

dimensions of performance Attributes of organizational performance that are related to organizations "doing the right things" (that is, appropriateness, availability, and efficacy) or organizations "doing things well" (continuity, effectiveness, efficiency, respect and caring, safety, and timeliness). All performance dimensions are definable, measurable, and improvable.

discrete variable A measurement that is limited to discrete options (for example, yes/no/unknown; less than or equal to 20 minutes/ greater than 20 minutes).

discrete variable indicator *See* rate-based indicator.

drug Any chemical compound that may be used on or administered to persons as an aid in the diagnosis, treatment, or prevention of disease or other abnormal condition.

drug administration   The act in which a prescribed dose of an identified drug is given to a patient.

drug dispensing   The issuance of one or more doses of a prescribed medication by a pharmacist or other authorized person to another person responsible for administering it.

drug error   *See* medication error.

eclampsia   The occurrence of one or more convulsions, or coma, not attributable to other cerebral conditions such as epilepsy or cerebral hemorrhage, in a patient with preeclampsia.

effectiveness   A performance dimension concerning the degree to which the care/intervention is provided in the correct manner, given the current state of knowledge, in order to achieve the desired/projected outcome(s) for the patient.

efficacy   A performance dimension concerning the degree to which the care/intervention used for the patient has been shown to accomplish the desired/projected outcome(s).

efficiency   A performance dimension referring to the ratio of the outcomes (results of care/intervention) for a patient to the resources used to deliver the care.

emphysema   A condition of the lung characterized by abnormal permanent enlargement of air spaces distal to the terminal bronchiole, accompanied by the destruction of their walls and with obvious fibrosis.

endometritis   Inflammation of the endometrium.

endotracheal intubation   The process of inserting an endotracheal tube into the trachea.

endotracheal tube   A tube passed into the trachea for administration of anesthesia, maintenance of an airway, aspiration of secretions, ventilation of the lungs, or prevention of entrance of foreign material, such as stomach contents, into the tracheobronchial tree.

expert   An individual who has acquired knowledge and/or experience pertinent to a specified function or process.

expert consensus   Agreement in opinion of experts.

expert panel or task force   A group of experts convened to accomplish an objective(s), such as a task force convened for indicator development.

external environment-based sources of performance variation   *See* variation, external environment-based sources of performance.

extrasystemic cause variation   *See* variation, special cause.

fishbone diagram   *See* cause-and-effect diagram.

flowchart   A pictorial summary that documents the steps, sequence, and relationship of the various operations involved in the performance of a function or a process.

flowcharting   The process of creating a flowchart for a function or a process.

function   A goal-directed, interrelated series of processes, such as patient assessment or information management functions.

function, important   An organizational function believed, on the basis of objective evidence or expert consensus, to increase the probability of desired patient health outcomes.

Glasgow Coma Scale (GCS)   An index to assess impairment of consciousness after head injury.

governing body   The individual(s), group, or agency that has ultimate authority and responsibility for establishing policy, maintaining patient care quality, and providing for organizational management and planning; other names for this group include the board, board of trustees, board of governors, and board of commissioners.

guideline, practice   Descriptive tool or standardized specification(s) for care of the typical patient in the typical situation, developed through a formal process that incorporates the best scientific evidence of effectiveness with expert opinion. Synonyms or near synonyms include clinical criteria, parameter (or practice parameter), protocol, algorithm, review criteria, preferred practice pattern, and guideline.

health care organization A generic term used to describe many types of organizations that provide health care services.

hospital A health care organization that has an organized medical staff and professional staff and inpatient facilities and provides medical, nursing, and related services for ill and injured patients. The definition of hospital varies among states and is based, for example, on a minimum number of beds and services that must be available to qualify as a hospital. Hospitals may be further specified by certain characteristics, resulting in such terms as accredited hospital, acute hospital, acute-care hospital, city hospital, community hospital, county hospital, federal hospital, for-profit hospital, government hospital, investor-owned hospital, mental health hospital, multihospital system, osteopathic hospital, nongovernment not-for-profit hospital, psychiatric hospital, rehabilitation hospital, teaching hospital, university hospital, and tertiary care hospital.

house staff Individuals, licensed as appropriate, who are graduates of medical, dental, osteopathic, or podiatric schools; who are appointed to a health care organization professional graduate training program that is approved by a nationally recognized accrediting body approved by the U.S. Department of Education; and who participate in patient care under the direction of licensed independent practitioners of the pertinent clinical disciplines who have clinical privileges in the organization and are members of, or are affiliated with, the medical staff.

human sensing *See* sensing.

ICD-9-CM *See International Classification of Diseases, Ninth Revision, Clinical Modification.*

IDES *See* Indicator Development Entry System.

IMS *See* indicator monitoring system.

independent practitioner *See* licensed independent practitioner.

indicator   1. A valid and reliable quantitative process or outcome measure related to one or more dimensions of performance such as effectiveness and appropriateness; 2. A statistical value that provides an indication of the condition or direction over time of an organization's performance of a specified process, or an organization's achievement of a specified outcome.

indicator, aggregate data   *See* aggregate data indicator.

indicator, continuous variable   *See* continuous variable indicator.

indicator, desirable   An outcome or a process indicator that measures a desirable activity or result of care, for example, patient survival.

indicator, discrete   *See* rate-based indicator.

indicator, outcome   An indicator that measures what happens or does not happen after a process, service, or activity is performed or not performed.

indicator, process   An indicator that measures an important, discrete care activity. The best process indicators focus on processes that are closely linked to patient outcomes, meaning that a scientific basis exists for believing that the process, when executed effectively, will increase the probability of a desired outcome.

indicator, rate-based   *See* rate-based indicator.

indicator, sentinel event   *See* sentinel event indicator.

indicator, undesirable   An outcome or a process indicator that measures an undesirable activity or result of care; for example, patient death or mortality.

indicator-based monitoring system   *See* indicator monitoring system.

Indicator Development Entry System (IDES)   Computer software and information management system permitting computerized aggregation of data elements for use by accredited health care organizations for independent self-analysis and to provide data elements for transfer to the Joint Commission for national comparative analysis during the beta phase of indicator testing.

Indicator Development Entry System logic The flow of general steps, according to precise aggregation rules, used to establish specific indicator occurrence rates from data elements in the Indicator Development Entry System.

indicator development form A form used to describe and record the development process for each indicator.

indicator-driven monitoring system *See* indicator monitoring system.

indicator monitoring system (IMS) A performance monitoring system designed to continuously collect objective data that are derived from the application of aggregate data indicators by health care organizations; aggregate, risk adjust as necessary, and analyze the performance data on a national level; provide comparative performance data to participating organizations for use in their internal performance improvement efforts; identify patterns that may call for more focused attention by the Joint Commission at the organizational level; and provide a national performance database that can serve as a resource for health services research.

indicator reliability The degree to which indicators accurately and completely identify occurrences from among all cases at risk of being indicator occurrences.

indicator testing process The process by which indicators are evaluated for many attributes including, for example, their degrees of reliability and validity, and their feasibility.

indicator underlying factors Patient-, practitioner-, organization systems'-, chance-, and environment-based characteristics that may explain variation in data and thereby direct performance improvement activities and efforts.

indicator validity The degree to which an indicator identifies events that merit further review by various individuals or groups providing or affecting the process or outcome defined by the indicator.

information Data that have been transformed through analysis and interpretation into a form useful for decision making.

International Classification of Diseases, Ninth Revision, Clinical Modification (ICD-9-CM)   The classification in current use for coding of morbidity and mortality of diagnoses and procedures; for indexing medical records by diagnoses and procedures; for compiling organization statistics; and for submitting claims to third-party payers. Published by the federal government.

laparotomy   An abdominal incision to gain access to the peritoneal cavity.

leaders, organization   The group of individuals that set expectations, develop plans, and implement procedures to assess and improve the quality of the organization's governance, management, clinical, and support processes. For example, leaders in hospitals include at least the leaders of the governing body; the chief executive officer and other senior managers; the elected and/or appointed leaders of the medical staff and the clinical departments and other medical staff in a hospital's administrative positions; and the nursing executive and other senior nursing leaders.

licensed independent practitioner   Any individual who is permitted by law and by the health care organization to provide patient care services without direction or supervision, within the scope of the individual's license, and in accordance with individually granted clinical privileges.

licensure   A legal right that is granted by a government agency in compliance with a statute governing an occupation (such as medicine or nursing) or the operation of an activity (such as a hospital).

mean   A measure of central tendency of a collection of data consisting of the sum of all the measurements of the data set divided by the total number of measurements in the data set; also called *average.*

measure   *See* measurement, performance measure, unit of measure.

measurement   1. The process of quantification; 2. The number resulting from the quantification process.

measurement data   Data resulting from the measurement process; forms one basis for performance assessment and improvement.

medical staff   An organizational body that has the overall responsibility for the quality of the professional services provided by individuals with clinical privileges and also the responsibility of accounting therefor to the governing body. The medical staff includes fully licensed physicians and may include other licensed individuals permitted by law and by the organization to provide patient care services independently (that is, without clinical direction or supervision) in the organization. Members have delineated clinical privileges that allow them to provide patient care services independently within the scope of their clinical privileges. Members and all others with individual clinical privileges are subject to medical staff and departmental bylaws and are subject to review as part of the organization's performance assessment and improvement activities.

medical staff credentialing   *See* credentialing.

medication   Any substance, whether a prescription or over-the-counter drug, that is taken orally or is injected, inserted, topically applied, or otherwise administered to a patient.

medication error   A discrepancy between what the physician ordered and what was reported to occur. Types of medication errors include: omission, unauthorized drug, extra dose, wrong dose, wrong dosage form, wrong rate, deteriorated drug, wrong administration technique, and wrong time. An omission type of medication error is the failure to give an ordered dose; a refused dose is not counted as an error if the nurse responsible for administering the dose tried to persuade the patient to take it but failed. Doses withheld according to written policies, such as for roentgenogram procedures, are not counted as omission errors. An unauthorized type of medication error is the administration of a dose of medication not authorized to be given to that patient. Instances of "brand or therapeutic substitution" are counted as unauthorized drug errors only where prohibited by institutional policy. A wrong dose type of medication error occurs when a patient receives an amount of medicine that is greater than or less than the amount ordered; the range of allowable deviation is based on hospital definition.

milestone   A meaningful event that marks completion of some aspect of a project.

minimum standard   The basic acceptable expectation of organizational performance; also refers to the one-page document titled "Minimum Standard" developed in 1919 by the American College of Surgeons in response to the need for a hospital standardization program.

morbidity and mortality conference   A medical staff conference, often department based, in which one or more cases are presented and reviewed. Cases may be presented and reviewed, for example, because they are unusual or complex, forced difficult management choices, or resulted in unexpected and undesirable outcomes. Discussions may cover many topics such as the value of new technologies, approaches to care that might have been employed, clinical findings that were overlooked, or an ethical dilemma presented by the case. Case conferences tend to be highly valued by clinicians as an effective method of learning. They are usually conducted in a nonjudgmental atmosphere and are considered clinically pertinent. They accord with medical training in that they often focus on individual cases.

myocardial infarction   *See* acute myocardial infarction.

neurologic deficit, peripheral   *See* peripheral neurologic deficit.

nondisease factors   Patient-based sources of performance variation, such as age, sex, and refusal of consent, that have an impact on care but that are not related to illness.

nosocomial infection   An infection acquired by a patient in a health care organization. The most common nosocomial infections are urinary tract infections, followed by surgical wound infections, pneumonia, and infections of the bloodstream.

nosocomial infection rate   The proportion describing the number of patients with nosocomial infection divided by the number of patients at risk of developing nosocomial infection. Rates may be stratified by taking into account certain patient factors that may predispose a specified group of patients to an increased risk of acquiring a nosocomial infection.

nurse, licensed practical/vocational An individual who is licensed by the state, commonwealth, or territory to provide basic nursing care under the supervision and direction of a registered nurse.

nurse, registered (RN) An individual who is qualified by an approved postsecondary program or baccalaureate or higher degree in nursing and licensed by the state, commonwealth, or territory to practice professional nursing.

objective 1. A term used to describe reality as it can be determined by observations made by individuals who are not experiencing the event; 2. Without bias or prejudice; 3. Something aimed at or striven for that is stated in measurable terms, has a specified time frame for achievement, and is related to the attainment of a goal.

organization *See* health care organization.

organizational performance *See* performance, organizational.

organization-based sources of performance variation *See* variation, organization-based sources of performance.

organization factor or organization-based factor An organization-related variable that may contribute to variation in performance data; usually is controllable by the organization and is the object of performance measurement and improvement processes.

outcome That which results from performance (or nonperformance) of a function(s) process(es). An outcome represents the cumulative effect of one or more processes on a patient at a defined point in time, as in patient survival (or death) following a medical intervention.

parenteral Not through the alimentary canal, but rather, by injection through some other route, such as subcutaneous, intramuscular, intraorbital, intracapsular, intraspinal, intrasternal, and intravenous.

patient   A person who has established a contractual relationship with a health care provider for that provider to render services or care to that person.

patient-based sources of performance variation   *See* variation, patient-based sources of performance.

patient factor or patient-based factor   An individual patient-related variable that may influence performance data; includes severity of illness, comorbid conditions, and nondisease factors. These factors usually are not within practitioners' or organizations' control.

patient health outcome   *See* outcome.

pattern   *See* data pattern.

percutaneous transluminal angioplasty   Dilatation of a blood vessel by means of a balloon catheter inserted through the skin and through the lumen of the vessel to the site of the narrowing, where the balloon is inflated to flatten plaque against the artery wall.

percutaneous transluminal coronary angioplasty (PTCA)   Dilatation of a coronary blood vessel by means of a balloon catheter inserted through the skin and through the lumen of the vessel to the site of the narrowing, where the balloon is inflated to flatten plaque against the artery wall.

performance   The way in which an individual, group, or organization carries out or accomplishes its important functions and processes.

performance, organizational   The way in which a health care organization carries out or accomplishes its important functions and processes; can be quantitatively measured and then compared with other measurements to make useful assessments. It incorporates a dimension of scale, meaning that there are levels of performance.

performance assessment   Involves, among other processes, analysis and interpretation of performance measurement data; the second segment of a performance measurement, assessment, and improvement system.

performance database   An organized comprehensive collection of data designed primarily to provide information concerning organizational and/or practitioner performance and the quality of patient care.

performance dimensions   *See* dimensions of performance.

performance improvement   The continuous study and adaptation of processes of providing health care services to increase the probability of achieving desired outcomes and to better meet the needs of patients and other users of services; the third segment of a performance measurement, assessment, and improvement system.

performance indicator   *See* indicator.

performance measure   Any device for measuring (quantifying) level of performance; also, an objective measure that may be used as an indicator of, say, quality.

performance measurement   The quantification of processes and outcomes using one or more dimensions of performance, such as availability and timeliness; the first segment of a performance measurement, assessment, and improvement system.

performance variation   *See* variation.

peripheral neurologic deficit   Functional defect, such as wrist drop, involving one or more peripheral nerves.

pharmacist   An individual who has a degree in pharmacy and is licensed to prepare, preserve, compound, and dispense drugs and chemicals.

physician   An individual who has received a degree of doctor of medicine or doctor of osteopathy and who is fully licensed to practice medicine.

physician licensure   The process by which a legal jurisdiction such as a state grants permission to a physician to practice medicine on finding that she or he has met acceptable qualification standards. Licensure also involves ongoing regulation of physicians by the legal jurisdiction, including the authority to revoke or otherwise restrict a physician's license to practice.

physician member of the medical staff A doctor of medicine or doctor of osteopathy who, by virtue of education, training, and demonstrated competence, is granted medical staff membership and clinical privileges by a health care organization to perform specified diagnostic or therapeutic procedures.

placenta previa A placenta that develops in the lower uterine segment, in the zone of dilatation, so that it covers or adjoins the internal os; painless hemorrhage in the last trimester, particularly during the eighth month, is the most common symptom.

policies and procedures The act, method, or manner of proceeding in some process or course of action; a particular course of action or way of doing something, such as policies and procedures governing the medical staff credentialing process.

practice guideline *See* guideline, practice.

practitioner-based sources of performance variation *See* variation, practitioner-based sources of performance.

practitioner factor or practitioner-based factor Individual practitioner-related variable that may contribute to variation in performance data; usually controllable and the object of a thorough monitoring process.

preeclampsia A toxemia of late pregnancy characterized by hypertension, edema, and proteinuria; when convulsions and coma are associated, it is called eclampsia.

process A goal-directed, interrelated series of actions, events, mechanisms, or steps.

process, important A process believed, on the basis of evidence or expert consensus, to increase the probability that desired outcomes will occur.

proportion *See* rate-based indicator.

provider, health care Health professional or health care organization, or group of health professionals or health care organizations, that provide health care services to patients.

quality of care The degree to which health services for individuals and populations increase the likelihood of desired health outcomes and are consistent with current professional knowledge.

quality improvement An approach to the continuous study and improvement of the processes of providing health care services to meet the needs of patients and others. Synonyms and near synonyms include continuous quality improvement (CQI), continuous improvement, organizationwide quality improvement, performance improvement, and total quality management (TQM).

quantification Determining that attribute of a thing by which it is greater or less than some other thing; assigning numbers to objects or events to describe their properties.

quantitative data Data expressed in specific measurement units.

rate-based indicator An aggregate data indicator in which the value of each measurement is expressed as a proportion or a ratio. In a proportion, the numerator is expressed as a subset of the denominator (for example, patients with cesarean section over all patients who deliver). In a ratio, the numerator and denominator measure different phenomena (for example, the number of patients with central lines who develop infections over central line days).

ratio *See* rate-based indicator.

registered nurse *See* nurse, registered.

reliability of indicator *See* indicator reliability.

reliability testing Quantification of the accuracy and completeness with which indicator occurrences are identified from among all cases at risk of being indicator occurrences.

respect and caring A performance dimension concerning the degree to which a patient, or designee, is involved in his or her own care decisions, and that those providing the services do so with sensitivity and respect for his or her needs and expectations and individual differences.

resuscitation, cardiopulmonary *See* cardiopulmonary resuscitation.

RN *See* nurse, registered.

safety A performance dimension concerning the degree to which the risk of an intervention and risk in the care environment are reduced for the patient and others, including the health care provider.

sensing The use of the senses (for example, sight, hearing) and memory as the sole bases on which to form conclusions and make decisions about observed phenomena.

sentinel event A serious event that requires further investigation each time it occurs.

sentinel event indicator A performance measure that identifies an individual event or phenomenon that always triggers further analysis and investigation and usually occurs infrequently and is undesirable in nature.

serum drug level Measured concentration of drug in serum or plasma.

severity of illness Patient-based sources of performance variation concerning the degree or stage of disease prior to treatment.

special care unit Organized service area with a concentration of qualified professional staff and supportive resources established to provide intensive care continuously on a 24-hour basis to critically ill patients. Such units include general intensive care, medical/surgical units, and other types of units that provide specialized intensive care (for example, burn and neonatal intensive care).

special cause A factor that sporadically induces variation over and above that inherent in the system; often appears as an extreme point or some specific, identifiable pattern in data.

special cause variation *See* variation, special cause.

special variation *See* variation, special cause.

systemic adjuvant therapy   Chemotherapy, hormonal/steroid therapy, biological response modifier therapy, or other systemic agents in addition to primary treatment by surgical resection and/or radiation therapy for cancer.

systemic cause variation   *See* variation, special cause.

task   The smallest measurable unit of work resulting in a predefined output.

task force   *See* expert panel.

threshold   The level or point at which a stimulus is strong enough to signal the need for organization response to indicator data and the beginning of the process of determining why the threshold has been approached or crossed.

timeliness   A performance dimension concerning the degree to which the care/intervention is provided to the patient at the time it is most beneficial or necessary.

total quality management   *See* quality improvement.

TQM   Abbreviation for total quality management; *see* quality improvement.

transportation services   The component of an organization responsible for the safe delivery of patients from one area to another.

trauma   Wound or injury.

trauma, blunt   Trauma due to nonpenetrating force that may occur as a result of a crushing injury, motor vehicle accident, fall, or assault with a blunt weapon.

trend   *See* data trend.

unit of measure   A defined amount of an attribute of a person, an activity, or a thing (such as an event, an object, or a phenomenon); for example, a Fahrenheit degree (a unit of measure) is a defined amount of the heat (an attribute) of an oven (an object).

utilization review   The examination and evaluation of the appropriateness of the use of resources of a health care organization.

vaginal birth after cesarean section (VBAC), attempted Trial of labor in a patient with a history of cesarean section or uterine scar from previous surgery as documented in the medical record.

vaginal birth after cesarean section (VBAC), failed Trial of labor resulting in delivery by repeat cesarean section.

vaginal birth after cesarean section (VBAC), successful Trial of labor resulting in vaginal delivery in a patient with a history of previous cesarean section.

validity of indicator *See* indicator validity.

validity testing Quantification of the extent to which an indicator identifies an event that merits further review by various individuals or groups providing or affecting the process or outcome defined by the indicator.

value A judgment based on the inverse relationship between the perceived quality of an organization's service and the cost of the service.

variation The inevitable difference among individual outputs of a process; excessive variation frequently leads to waste and loss, such as the occurrence of undesirable patient health outcomes and increased cost of health services. Sources of performance variation are patient based, practitioner based, organization based, chance based, and external environment based. Types of variation include common cause and special cause.

variation, assignable cause *See* variation, special cause.

variation, attributable cause *See* variation, special cause.

variation, chance A source of variation due solely to chance or happenstance.

variation, common cause A source of variation that is always present and is part of the random variation inherent in all processes. Its origin can usually be traced to an element of the system only management can correct.

variation, external environment-based sources of performance Factors, such as number of nursing beds available in the community, that are typically outside of an organization's control but with which an organization must cope.

variation, extrasystemic cause *See* variation, special cause.

variation, organization-based sources of performance Factors that are usually within an organization's control and influence the underlying average effectiveness of care the organization provides.

variation, patient-based sources of performance Factors usually outside of an organization's or a practitioner's control, which influence the underlying average risk the patient carries on admission. Includes severity of illness, comorbid conditions, and nondisease factors that may have an impact on care.

variation, performance *See* variation.

variation, practitioner-based sources of performance Factors usually within an organization's control that influence the type of assessments and treatments patients may receive and the effectiveness of those assessments and treatments.

variation, special cause A source of variation that is intermittent, unpredictable, and unstable. It is not inherently present in a system; rather, it arises from causes that are not part of the system as designed. It tends to cluster by person, place, and time, and it should be eliminated by an organization if it results in undesirable outcomes.

variation, systemic cause *See* variation, common cause.

VBAC *See* vaginal birth after cesarean section, attempted.

Index